PATIENT EXPECTATIONS

PATIENT EXPECTATIONS

How Economics, Religion, and Malpractice Shaped
Therapeutics in Early America

CATHERINE L. THOMPSON

UNIVERSITY OF MASSACHUSETTS PRESS
Amherst and Boston

Copyright © 2015 by University of Massachusetts Press
All rights reserved
Printed in the United States of America

ISBN 978-1-62534-159-4 (paperback); 158-7 (hardcover)

Designed by Sally Nichols
Set in Adobe Garamond Pro
Printed and bound by Maple Press, Inc.

Library of Congress Cataloging-in-Publication Data

Thompson, Catherine L. (Catherine Lynne), 1962– , author.
Patient expectations : how economics, religion, and malpractice shaped therapeutics in early America / Catherine L. Thompson.
p. ; cm.
Includes bibliographical references and index.
ISBN 978-1-62534-159-4 (pbk. : alk. paper) — ISBN 978-1-62534-158-7 (hardcover : alk. paper)
I. Title.
[DNLM: 1. Attitude to Health—United States. 2. Patient Participation—history—United States. 3. History, 18th Century—United States. 4. History, 19th Century—United States. 5. Patient Care—history—United States. 6. Physician's Practice Patterns—history—United States. W 85]
R728
610.68—dc23

2015009307

British Library Cataloguing-in-Publication Data
A catalogue record for this book is available from the British Library.

*To My Heroes,
Robert N. Thompson
and
Cornelia H. Dayton*

CONTENTS

Acknowledgments	ix
Introduction	1
1. Medical Practice in Massachusetts	9
2. Self-Medication in the Nineteenth Century	33
3. Money and Medicine	49
4. Patient Expectations and Religious Beliefs	67
5. Medicine and Malpractice	92
Conclusion	113
Tables	117
Appendix A. Self-Medication Data	137
Appendix B. Diagnosis Tables for the 1820s, 1830s, and 1840s	139
Appendix C. List of Massachusetts Cases Identified	149
Appendix D. Criminal Cases in Massachusetts	152
Appendix E. Methodologies Used	153
Notes	155
Index	185

ACKNOWLEDGMENTS

I am continually amazed at the time and effort people are willing to dedicate to me. I thank Cornelia H. Dayton, Richard D. Brown, and Christopher Clark for devoting their time, expertise, and support. I extend special thanks to Patrick Blythe, Dominic DeBrincat, and Michael Neagle, my writing club; to my anonymous readers, who exemplified the concept of constructive criticism; and to Alan Swedlund, Conrad Wright, and Robert A. Gross, who provided guidance. Finally, I thank the editing staff, especially Clark Dougan, at the University of Massachusetts Press for their patience and humor.

I am grateful for the funding provided by several institutions during the early stages of this project. A fellowship from the University of Connecticut Humanities Institute allowed me to devote a full year to writing. The Francis A. Countway Fellowship at the Boston Medical Library and the Massachusetts General Hospital gave me their time and access to their nineteenth-century hospital records. The Andrew W. Mellon Fellowship at the Massachusetts Historical Society funded several weeks of research in an archive rich with sources. The Kate B. and Hall J. Peterson Fellowship provided me with the opportunity to spend a glorious summer month at the American Antiquarian Society as well as to receive the advice of the staff and other resident fellows. The Francis C. Wood Institute Fellowship made possible a research visit to the College of Physicians in Philadelphia.

PATIENT EXPECTATIONS

INTRODUCTION

Employed as a pharmaceutical representative for nine years, I sat in many a clinician's waiting room passing the time by talking to patients. Over the years, I began to see the medical profession through their eyes. I witnessed many instances of how patients' demands, fears, and lifestyles influenced their medical care. So when beginning my research for this book, I came to the project curious about the extent to which patients have shaped medical practice throughout history. I was particularly interested in the major shift that took place in medical therapeutics in the early nineteenth century. Historians have offered a variety of explanations for this change, but primarily from the point of view of physicians. I wanted to see how our understanding of this period might change if medical therapeutics were viewed through the eyes of patients.

The medical history of the early American Republic is quite well documented. Late-eighteenth- and early-nineteenth-century doctors followed a course of treatment, often referred to as "heroic" depletive therapy, that was characterized by puking, purging, and bleeding. Dr. Benjamin Rush was one of the most prominent and influential proponents of this approach. A signer of the Declaration of Independence, medical school professor, and prolific writer, Rush became renowned during the 1793 yellow fever epidemic in Philadelphia, when he prescribed large doses of purgatives and copious bleeding as cures. He quickly publicized his methods, advocating calomel and bloodletting as a panacea or cure for all ills.[1]

Based on a theory of "humors" dating back to Galen (129–ca. 210),[2] Rush's heroic style had a major impact on American medical practice throughout the first half of the nineteenth century. His medical training in Edinburgh shaped his approach to medical treatment. Drawing on the theories of Herman Boerhaave, William Cullen, and his fellow student John Brown, Rush believed that the circulatory system held the key to human health, and that debility, in which strong stimuli exhausted the body, was the cause of illness.[3] He therefore recommended copious depletion in order to rid the body of harmful stimuli and bring it back into balance.

During the 1820s and 1830s Rush's theories came under increasing criticism. A new medical movement arose, contributing to a shift in medical practice. American doctors who had trained in Paris rejected the theoretical predilections of Rush and other heroic practitioners in favor of the "empirical pursuit of truth . . . rooted in the collection of observed facts."[4] Empiricists advocated observation over deduction, the application of scientific method with a trained eye developed through experiences at the bedside, in hospital wards, and in autopsy rooms.[5] Believing that certain diseases were self-limiting and would run their course naturally, they practiced an expectant method of treatment, encouraging physicians to take a wait-and-see attitude. If illness persisted, they sought to guide the recovery with mild therapeutics, dietary recommendations, exercise if appropriate, and change in environmental factors if necessary. Over time a growing number of doctors embraced empiricism, until by midcentury the theories and practices that had long dominated American medicine had been largely discredited.

Many explanations for the change in therapeutic practice have been proposed, including public outcry over the barbaric measures of heroic therapies, increased medical competition, and new medical theories. Whatever the causes, orthodox physicians were forced to rethink their therapeutic approaches.[6] In *The Therapeutic Perspective,* John Harley Warner found sharp regional differences in medical practice, showing that not all American practitioners treated with heroic doses. Yet his study focuses on hospital wards rather than medical practices in the home, where most people were treated; it does not establish whether these regional differences occurred in the day-to-day practice of medicine. Although scholars differ on whether this transition was gradual or abrupt and on whether regional differences in the use of heroic therapies were significant, they are consistent in telling the story from the point of view of medical professionals.[7]

In short, what medical histories have tended to overlook is the role played by patients in shaping medical practice. At its core, this book uses diaries, correspondence, and account books of nineteenth-century Massachusetts physicians and patients to explore private medical practice, and ultimately to demonstrate that this is not the story of a dramatic rise and fall in the use of heroic therapy but of a gradual shift in patients' expectations of medical care. Patients did not endure horrific treatments for decades only to abandon them suddenly in favor of alternative practices. To begin with, Massachusetts doctors never used heroic depletive therapies to the extent that many medical historians have suggested. Many patients' journals and correspondence recorded satisfaction with the treatments they received. By the mid-nineteenth century, changes in economics, religious beliefs, and the law affected expectations of medical care. These changes contributed to an increasing dissatisfaction with orthodox therapies among specific patient groups, who no longer simply sought just palliative care but instead demanded complete eradication of disease. A shift in patient expectations, then, provides a clearer understanding of why medical therapeutics changed over the course of the early nineteenth century.

By repositioning patients as active shapers rather than passive recipients of their medical care, this book challenges standard accounts of the evolution of American medicine. My study begins with the 1750s, before the ascendency of heroic therapeutics, and ends in 1860, with a new approach to treatment on the rise and the recently formed American Medical Association (1847) in the process of establishing a cohesive medical profession. Although limited to Massachusetts, the evidence I examine is drawn from different parts of the Commonwealth—Boston and surrounding towns, towns of Worcester County in the central part of the state, and Deerfield in the west. This regional variation, demographic as well as geographical, provides the framework for a comparative analysis of patients' diaries, physicians' account books and papers, and other medical documents.[8] Boston, as the largest regional commercial port and the home of a premier medical school (Harvard, founded in 1782), served as one of the main medical centers of the young United States. Evidence drawn from private practice in Boston differs in some aspects from what John Harley Warner found in the wards of the Massachusetts General Hospital (MGH), while data on Worcester and Deerfield reveal variations in therapeutic approach between urban and rural communities.

I focus on relationships between patients and orthodox physicians (those who received training through medical school or apprenticeship and who practiced in a manner widely accepted by their peers). The unorthodox practitioners (those who had received no training or practiced approaches not widely accepted by the majority of practitioners) are examined only in terms of how they interacted with patients and orthodox practitioners.[9] I do not consider surgical practice because, as Warner states, "at least through the 1860s the mechanical aspects of surgical therapeutics (though not its medical ones) held an epistemological status fundamentally different from that occupied by *medical* therapeutics."[10] In other words, there existed standard surgical precepts that were applied to all surgical patients, whereas medical therapeutics, governed by a dependence on the patient and the environment (called specificity), differed from patient to patient.

Nor does this analysis address epidemics. Massachusetts physicians kept separate records for the duties they performed during epidemics, suggesting that data gathered during epidemics was fundamentally different from the recurrent trials of personal illness. Sicknesses were common and expected; epidemics brought fear and panic. The practices I examine in this study would today fall within the purview of internal medicine. The ailments most often treated included gastrointestinal ailments, fevers, rheumatism, lung problems, skin diseases, cuts, and wounds.

The chapters are arranged around various elements that challenge commonly held notions of medical practice in the Early Republic. The first chapter looks at the frequency of use of purges, pukes, and bleeding in private medical practice. With a comparative analysis of medical account books using a 10 percent random sampling, I consider five Massachusetts physicians who practiced medicine from the 1780s to the 1830s to determine the use of various therapeutic drugs. Based on an extensive database of physicians' daybooks that I created, this chapter analyzes urban and rural private practice to reveal how patients experienced and influenced therapeutics. Two physicians, Moses Mosman, who lived near Boston, and William Williams of Deerfield, practiced during most of the period studied. Their lengthy tenures as town physicians provide us an opportunity to gauge the extent to which medical theories influenced individual practitioners' therapeutic habits over time. In the end, what we learn is that whether a physician prescribed medicines or not, and what kind, depended in important ways on his patients' expectations. Physicians' casebooks and patients' journals recount negotiations between doctors and patients that determined individual treatments. These physicians' prescribing habits reveal that they rarely employed harsh cathartics and emetics during the supposedly peak-period use of heroic therapeutics and that most patients consulted physicians for pain and constipation, expressing satisfaction with treatments they received.

In addition, patients could and did obtain remedies themselves. Then, as now, over-the-counter drugs constituted a large lucrative business, as evidenced by common newspaper advertisements offering a range of products available for self-medication. In chapter 2, an examination of patients' diaries highlights how many patients self-medicated and consulted professional healers simultaneously. Physicians' journals and hospital records from the MGH record doctors' reactions to their patients' use of other remedies and complicate impressions that orthodox physicians had combative relations with unorthodox practitioners. In many instances, interaction and sometimes congenial cooperation between diverse groups of practitioners can be seen. Intake interviews of patients offer an unusual glimpse into working-class men's and women's self-medication patterns. Contradicting images of patients as passive recipients of harsh medical treatment by physicians, data suggest that patients were just as, or more, likely to dose themselves with calomel and emetics than physicians were to prescribe them.

The first two chapters demonstrate that Massachusetts physicians did not practice heroic depletive therapy to the extent described in most medical histories and that patients frequently expressed satisfaction with their treatments in their correspondence and journals. Yet public attitudes toward orthodox medicine did change by the 1830s, and the change was primarily attributable to different patient expectations. Several factors influenced what people expected of medical care, including the economic practices of physicians. In chapter 3, I examine data from account books of physicians who practiced from the 1760s to the 1850s that reveal a shift in direction toward cash payments for medical treatment rather than payment in goods and services. This pattern was not uniform, however. Payment in cash occurred primarily in eastern and central Massachusetts, whereas western medical practices remained relatively unchanged.

Economic changes in patient–physician relationships exacerbated inequities in medical choices among different patient populations. The social ramifications of the movement toward cash payments affected specific patient populations differently. Middle-class groups benefited. No longer entangled in the complicated web of credit and debit, they pursued cure or relief from a variety of practitioners. Conversely, less wealthy patients, who were denied credit and had little cash, could no longer pay promptly or in forms that were acceptable. Thus, they were forced to seek medical care from public institutions like hospitals and charitable organizations, limiting their control over their health care.

Hospitals, such as MGH, that offered minimal comforts in the wards nevertheless provided rest, warmth, and caretaking that were sometimes unavailable, impractical, or problematic at home. Domestics and immigrants often lived in boardinghouses that did not have warm beds or people to care for them and contained other persons to infect—all reasons to seek care in a hospital ward. Despite popular notions, hospitals were not always places of last resort. This applied to the middle class but not to lower-class patients who could no longer barter for private home care. For those who were suffering from chronic diarrhea or dyspepsia, the hospital could be the first choice after self-medication. Both health treatises and experience had made it clear that these symptoms could be early signs of typhus, typhoid, or dysentery. Such diseases could kill if rest, proper diet, and care were not found quickly. Records from the MGH confirm that the likelihood of a patient seeking care in a hospital was not just a function of income or ability to pay in cash or type of ailment; age, nationality, marital status, gender, social credit, and length of residency all could be factors in the decision to enter a hospital.

Chapter 4 demonstrates how shifts in the religious landscape in Massachusetts influenced patients' attitudes toward illness and medical practice. In the eighteenth century, Congregationalists believed that, while some illnesses had natural causes, others could be instances of God testing or preparing their souls. Patients filled diaries, journals, and letters expressing their anxieties over whether their illnesses were natural or God's messages to them (called "special providences"). Seasonal epidemics, a high number of infant deaths, and industrial accidents constantly reminded patients in the Early Republic of their mortality. Late-eighteenth- and early-nineteenth-century people coped in many ways, including prayer. They prayed for God's guidance and accepted His will; this served as their way of exerting control over seemingly random events.

Over the course of the nineteenth century, the popularization of science did not translate into a decline in piety but rather into an increase in religious pluralism. Many patients sought control both in spirituality and in scientific pursuits. The language of cure reflects this. "Cure" came to connote not just relief from suffering but the eradication of the disease itself. The expectation that illness could and should be completely cured bolstered patients' confidence in the possibility of saving their bodies as well as their souls. Any person could avoid illness by living rightly, both spiritually and physically.

Different religious denominations debated how to achieve this goal. Unitarians looked outward. For them, the reform of society and individuals held the answer. Transcendentalists believed that God had equipped each human being inwardly with the proper conscience to live piously. Illness came when one wandered too far from one's divine intuition. Since illness arose from a man's choices, then perhaps a cure could be found through them as well. Revivalists still looked to God's direct guidance, but no longer waited passively for conversion: participants actively sought to be saved and healed. Medical expectations did not change as a result of secularization but because patients refused to be victimized by the caprices of disease without taking action themselves. A focus on changing the temporal world became a tool to achieve both salvation and good health; *this* was God's will.

Chapter 5 explores changes in legal understandings of malpractice and its intersection with patient expectations. Medical malpractice suits provide clear evidence of patients' dissatisfaction with the care they had received. Analysis of these suits shows the influence of patient expectations on a critical change in the legal understanding of a physician's duty to patients—a shift from nuisance to negligence. Before 1835, malpractice cases were rare and usually involved surgeries that had resulted in deformity or death. In *Medical Malpractice in Nineteenth-century America,* Kenneth DeVille argues that malpractice cases surged after 1835 and began to involve other types of medical cases. DeVille based his conclusion on appellate cases, which may not be representative of most malpractice cases.[11] Little scholarship exists on malpractice suits in the lower courts. An analysis of thirty-one cases in both lower and appeal courts in Massachusetts exposes factors that contributed to the rise in malpractice suits as well as the motives of patients who sued.

With the advent of industrialization, patient–physician relationships mirrored a broader trend of employer–employee relations in urban centers. Before the nineteenth century, employers had often provided care during illnesses or incapacitation due to injury on the job. As industrialization progressed, employers became less benevolent toward employees, and work injuries were no longer handled informally but through lawsuits. Eventually, physicians and patients came to view malpractice suits in the context of general negligence. Physicians continued to argue that they should not be held to the standards of an increasingly complicated medical profession, whereas juries saw it differently. If doctors could demand payment in cash or notes as tradesmen did, then patients could demand that physicians be held to same standards as tradesmen. Patients expected to be cured by doctors, especially as God became decreasingly linked with the causes of illness. Judges saw malpractice suits within an even broader context of public policy: no longer did they base the outcomes of suits on individual circumstances, but in terms of what was best for society. The rise of malpractice suits highlights conflicting legal views of patient–physician relationships.

When we position patients as active participants in their own health care, changes in patient expectations offer a fuller explanation of an important transition in medical history. Specifically, when we examine three important societal influences—economic practices, religious beliefs, and the rise of malpractice suits—patients emerge not as objects of medical practices but as active participants in a medical relationship that was at once commercial and intimate. Through an analysis of patient expectations, we begin to understand the roles played by different patient populations as shapers of medical products and services. This work does not constitute an exhaustive study of what influenced patients in making their medical choices and in forming their expectations of medical care; individual variations and life experiences make this impossible. However, when using economics, religion, and law to understand an interactive relationship between patients and their physicians at the ground level, what emerges is a picture of medical care that was not altered as much by medical theory or medical competition as it was by changing patient expectations.

1
Medical Practice in Massachusetts

In one of his children's books, author Francis C. Woodworth reminisced for his young readers about his childhood physician, Dr. Windham. In *A Peep at Our Neighbors* (1852), Woodworth described Windham as a doctor who "went to work at his patient, as a priest of a darker age would go to work at one supposed to be possessed of a devil." Woodworth complained of Windham using the "contents of half the vials in his saddle-bags on us, to say nothing of the blood which flowed from our veins at the tap of his lancet."[1] Woodworth's portrayal of his real or imagined childhood doctor provides just one of many examples of increasing criticisms of heroic depletive therapy by the mid-nineteenth century.

Benjamin Rush receives much of the credit for Windham's tortuous therapeutic approach. Oliver Wendell Holmes, Sr., lamented in 1860 about what he viewed as Rush's harmful influence on medical practice early in the century. Holmes counseled as follows: if a student wished "to understand the tendencies of the American medical mind . . . I would make him read the life and writings of Benjamin Rush," whom Holmes credited with giving "a direction to the medical mind of the country more than any other one man."[2] Historians of medicine have similarly noted Rush's impact on nineteenth-century medicine. Of Rush, one scholar states: "During the last two decades of his life, his heroic style would have a major impact on American practice, and it would remain significant, if somewhat less influential, well beyond 1850."[3] Standard therapeutic narratives further describe how in the 1820s heroic therapy came under attack from competing medical sects, such as the Thomsonians and homeopaths, and within the ranks of traditionally trained physicians, namely the empiricists who practice the expectant method of therapy.[4] As public and professional criticism increased, the use of the heroic regimen decreased.

Data compiled from physicians' account books in Massachusetts challenge this view of medicine in the Early Republic. Private practitioners in Massachusetts from the 1790s through the 1820s never practiced heroic depletive therapy rigorously, suggesting that standard narratives overstate Rush's influence on medical treatments beyond Philadelphia. Patient diaries and physicians' records show that, at least in Massachusetts, patients were satisfied with their therapeutic treatments in the late eighteenth and early nineteenth centuries. When medical practice did shift to a more expectant approach after the 1820s, it did so in response to changing patient expectations.

Furthermore, an investigation of whether heroic methods such as bleeding and purging began to decrease in the 1820s shows geographical disparities among private practitioners. John H. Warner's study explores the use of heroic remedies in hospital wards. He found that whether or not physicians in a specific region continued to practice heroic medicine after 1820 depended on how medical professionals derived their professional identities. In Boston, identities were derived from social and institutional connections rather than largely from practice. Thus, Boston physicians practicing at the Massachusetts General Hospital (MGH) decreased their practice of bloodletting and dispensing calomel between the 1820s and 1850s, embracing the expectant approach to medical treatment. Doctors at the Commercial Hospital of Cincinnati (CHC), however, felt more insecure when faced with criticism and continued to dose with mercury and treat via venesection.[5] Warner's work suggests that therapeutics were "subject to sharp regional and even personal variation." Because Warner's study focuses on hospital wards rather than private practice, one historian concluded that "unfortunately, we do not know enough about actual clinical practice (as distinct from theory) in the late eighteenth and early nineteenth centuries to characterize shifts in therapeutics with much accuracy or certitude."[6] Study of physicians in Massachusetts demonstrates that doctors rarely implemented heroic approaches in their private practice and that differences between urban and rural practices emerged after the 1820s.

Patients' diaries and doctors' casebooks record anecdotal data that verify a trend toward an expectant approach found in the MGH. Mary Lowell documented in her diary in September 1843 that she had kept her daughter Georgina home from school due to severe stomach cramps. "I thought she was going to have the complaint of the season," Lowell wrote, fearing that her daughter had contracted the typhus fever that had befallen many of her friends. She sent for a Dr. Adams, "who seemed to think the trouble would pass off, as it has, without medicine."[7] Adams, a Boston physician, practiced the expectant method. He waited to see if Georgina's body would fight off the disease before intervening.[8]

Dr. Joseph Sargent of Worcester provides another example of expectant therapy. Sargent consulted Dr. James Jackson, Sr. (who practiced at MGH), regarding his patient, Samuel O. Spunn. Sargent was concerned by "a collection of crude tubercles in both sides at the upper part" of his patient's lungs. Jackson advised him to have the patient "resort to a warmer climate to escalate the changes of the spring." He also counseled abstinence from medicines.[9] Physicians' casebooks and patients' diaries provide glimpses of a de-emphasis on heroic therapy in Massachusetts private practice. To discover with more precision what change, if any, there was in therapeutic treatments requires a study of physicians' account books and daybooks.[10] From such an analysis a clearer picture of what remedies physicians used to treat their patients in private practice and how patients shaped medical treatment emerges.

With a comparative analysis of medical account books using a 10 percent random sampling, I studied five physicians' account books in order to determine the use of various therapeutic drugs. The analysis indicates that neither contemporary public criticism nor historical characterizations of American medicine as dominated by heroic depletive therapy describe actual medical practice in Massachusetts. Excessive bloodletting and purging with calomel—primary agents of heroic therapy—never occurred in the medical practices in Boston, Worcester, and Deerfield under scrutiny here, confirming that contemporary and historical characterizations of medicine during this period as harsh and barbaric are exaggerated.[11]

Criteria for the selection of account books analyzed included consistent documentation of patient name and treatments given at each visit. Five physicians' account books were chosen to establish prescribing habits from 1763 to 1838 clinical practices located in Boston and Sudbury in eastern Massachusetts, Worcester and Ashburnham in the central part of the state, and Deerfield in the west. By using a computer-generated, randomized numbers list in which each number corresponded to an entry of the patient's name and treatments prescribed, I compiled a database of treatments for each doctor.[12] In this manner, a comparison of the five physicians' prescribing habits in three different periods—before 1790, 1790 to 1820, and after 1820 was possible. The prescribing patterns before 1790 demonstrate compounds dispensed before heroic medicine allegedly became popular among physicians. The period 1790 to 1820 marked the height of heroic therapeutics usage, according to historians of medicine. After 1820, heroic therapy began to decline. The use of primary agents of heroic therapy such as bloodletting, calomel, Ipecacuanha (a strong emetic), tartar emetic, and opiates provides the most direct index of physicians who aggressively practiced heroic depletive therapy.[13] Thus, I analyzed the account books in this project for use of calomel and other cathartics, emetics, opiates or narcotics, and bloodletting to ascertain the extent to which these five physicians were practicing heroic medicine. A high incidence of "no medicine prescribed" as well as a lack of or low use of heroic remedies suggest a practitioner who adopted the expectant approach to medicine.

Of the five physicians, Moses Mosman (1742–1817) of Sudbury, near Boston, practiced medicine the longest—fifty-four years. It is unclear with whom Mosman apprenticed. His account books survive for the years 1763 to 1817.[14] They reveal a physician who practiced medicine conservatively and with a variety of remedies; no ingredient surpassed the 12 percent mark of his total prescriptions, and the majority never accounted for more than 2 percent (see tables 1.1 and 1.2).[15]

Abraham Lowe (1775–1834) of Ashburnham, in Worcester County, practiced for nearly fifty years. He served one year in the American Revolution as a "common soldier" and commenced three years of study under Abraham Haskell of Lunenburg in 1780. Lowe was the sole physician in his town for most of the years of his practice. The author of his obituary described him as a "judicious physician" and praised him for his obstetric abilities. Lowe's membership in the Massachusetts Medical Society identifies him as an orthodox physician, as do his prescribing habits, such as his use of calomel (see table 1.3).[16]

William Stoddard Williams (1762–1829) practiced medicine in Deerfield from 1785 to 1828. Williams served as a medical apprentice under his father, Thomas. He furthered his medical education with an apprenticeship served under Erastus Sergeant of West Stockbridge for two years, from 1781 to 1783. Like his father, Williams became an active member in the community, serving as justice of the peace beginning in 1814.[17] Williams left twenty-eight volumes of detailed account books documenting his medical visits and prescriptions. Three were chosen for analysis; they show a physician who practiced orthodox medicine (see tables 1.4–1.6)[18]

Stephen West Williams (1790–1855), like his father William and grandfather Thomas before him, enjoyed a long medical practice in Deerfield.[19] Unlike his familial predecessors, Stephen went to medical school, graduating from King's College (now Columbia University) with an MD degree before serving an apprenticeship with his father. He lectured at the Berkshire Medical Institute on medical law and published several articles in scientific and medical journals. As a noted historian, he wrote a book on his most famous ancestor, the Reverend John Williams, who was held captive during the famous Deerfield Indian raid in 1704.[20] Stephen's account books, spanning the years 1836–38, depict a physician who used a smaller array of drugs than his father did, reflecting the prescribing habits of many orthodox physicians of his time (see table 1.7).

Caleb Hopkins Snow's (1796–1835) records offer a window into therapeutics in Boston during the 1820s. He received a medical degree from Brown University in 1821 after graduating with a bachelor's degree there in 1813 and serving as a librarian from 1814 to 1818. After medical school, he returned to his native Boston and set up a large, prosperous practice. Like Stephen Williams, he wrote several books, including *History of Boston with Some Account of its Environs* (1825).[21] Snow's ledger exemplifies the prescribing habits of a physician who had embraced the expectant approach to medicine (see table 1.8).

By comparing the physicians' prescribing patterns in key therapeutic categories—bloodletting, calomel, cathartics, emetics, opiates, and how often one chose not to prescribe medicine at all—possible explanations for each physician's therapeutic choices can be considered. Negotiations between patients and their physicians (as much as public criticisms of medical practice or shifts in medical theory) provide many explanations for the remedies prescribed. Interestingly, none of the five physicians ever embraced heroic therapeutics to the degree Benjamin Rush did or in ways that were criticized in mid-nineteenth-century print.

Bloodletting represents a common practice in heroic therapeutics. Venesection, wet cupping, scarification, and leeches represent the most common methods of bloodletting in the Early Republic.[22] Doctors used leeching and cupping to relieve pain and inflammation in localized areas. To treat fevers, physicians employed venesection. Publicly, orthodox physicians became associated with aggressive bloodletting from the late eighteenth century to the mid-nineteenth century. Some physicians who eschewed frequent or copious bleeding were categorized as practitioners of the expectant approach to medicine. At MGH, physicians practicing in the hospital decreased their use of bloodletting. In the 1830s hospital records show that bloodletting was used 35 percent of the time; that number dropped to 22 percent in the 1840s, and to 14 percent in the 1850s.[23]

The five practitioners in this study never bled their patients as much as the physicians at MGH.[24] In his Sudbury practice, Mosman only documented bleeding 2 percent of the time from 1786 to 1793, and that infrequent resort to the heroic procedure remained unchanged from 1802 to 1820 (see table 1.9). He does not appear to have bled his patients much either before the "heroic" era or during the height of its popularity. In the more rural areas of Ashburnham and Deerfield, the analysis of Lowe's and William Williams's prescribing habits produced similar results. William Williams in Deerfield recorded bleeding his patients in 5 percent of the entries from 1786 to 1791, 2 percent from 1804 to 1806, and 4 percent from 1825 to 1828. In the 1830s, when heroic depletive therapy found harsh critics, Stephen Williams bled patients at the low rate of his father—3 percent from 1836 to 1838. Boston physician Snow's records from 1827 to 1828 indicate that he bled his patients less than 1 percent of the time (see table 1.9). Not one of these physicians studied was influenced by the heroic therapeutic trend of frequent bleeding from the 1790s through the 1820s.[25]

Of course, it is possible that bloodletting was so fundamental or so common that Massachusetts physicians in private practice simply did not always bother to record having prescribed it. Yet all five physicians consistently recorded their treatments. Lowe and William Williams were particularly meticulous in documenting their visits, prescriptions, and charges; they rarely entered the generic expressions "and sundry meds" or "visit and meds" (see the "Meds, not specified" category in table 1.11). In other words, their documentation appears to be fairly precise and complete. Another explanation of bleeding's low incidence may lie in the fact that patients often bled themselves and thus perhaps felt no need to pay a physician to do so.

Indications of frequent self-bleeding appeared in printed health guides such as James Parkinson's *Medical Admonitions* (1803). On fevers, Parkinson complained that many persons seemed willing to depend on "the recommendation of some ignorant, but well meaning friend" to propose a cure. "Thus, bleeding is often had recourse to, immediately on appearance of fever, it being the popular opinion, that bleeding is the most effective means of removing that disease." Parkinson rejected the use of bleeding to treat fevers as was the practice of many patients, as he believed that fevers were seldom cured in this way.[26] Parkinson's advice stressed that bleeding should be carried out only under professional guidance.

Patient diaries also offer evidence of self-bloodletting. Deborah Fiske depended on leeching so much to relieve her inflammation that "she learned to apply these treatments herself, to the point of raising her own leeches."[27] Perhaps Fiske did not require bleeding by a physician because she frequently applied leeches to treat her inflammation. Self-application of leeches or the opening of veins for small quantities of blood (both examples of bloodletting) may have been prevalent, but copious bleeding could prove dangerous and thus was understood to require professional assistance. This may also explain why patients at MGH were bled more than patients in private practice. Physicians at MGH bled more frequently because their patients were seriously ill, motivating doctors to use more aggressive approaches.

Massachusetts private practitioners may not have bled often, but data from physicians' records demonstrate that doctors persisted in bloodletting well into the nineteenth century. Joseph Sargent's 1840 medical records show that he continued to apply leeches and practice venesection on his patients. One example involved his treatment of a forty-four-year-old for inflammation and pain in his urethra after the man had had an evening in which he "had connexion c/ [with an] unknown woman." Sargent proceeded to apply four leeches to the hernia he found in lower groin area. The doctor then gave his patient a dose of sulfate of magnesia (a mild cathartic) and directed him to follow a liquid and vegetable diet as well as to bath his penis three times a day in cold vinegar and water. After nearly a month of the repeated application of leeches for two to three hours at a time, the peddler was able to achieve a slight erection.[28] Many patients expressed their satisfaction and relief after bloodletting, as documented by Sargent.

Stephen Williams explained why physicians continued to bleed patients well into the mid-nineteenth century. He stated that bleeding was "more temperately used, and its services in highly acute inflammation are still considered to be invaluable."[29] In other words, by the mid-nineteenth century Massachusetts physicians rarely bled as frequently or copiously (if they ever did) as Rush advocated for fevers and other afflictions.[30] Instead, they used bloodletting for local inflammation.

Although Massachusetts physicians did not deserve such ridicule themselves, they must have been aware of the public criticism the orthodox medical profession received for the practice of bleeding patients. Printed works that ridiculed the practice abounded among treatises written by homeopaths and other medical sects, as well as in literature. For example, *Barn-yard Rhymes,* a poem about a turkey, goose, duck, and cock that mocked all nineteenth-century medical practices, contained this verse on Mr. Gobbler's experience of bleeding:

> And what I suffered, first and last,
> 'Twould make your feathers stand aghast . . .
> Every third day I was bled,
> All to ease my lungs he said.
> I soon was brought to skin and bone,
> And fairly on my beam ends thrown.
> But, thanks to a good constitution,
> I weathered through his persecution;
> Glad to escape with nothing worse
> Than weakness and an empty purse.[31]

Poems and cartoons depicted practitioners of heroic medicine as constantly torturing patients by bleeding and purging them. Only those with a strong constitution could weather such persecution.

Massachusetts physician Jacob Porter revealed his awareness of Rush's methods, and he appeared to be uncomfortable bleeding frequently and copiously. In an April 1810 passage of Porter's casebook, he wrote that his mother-in-law had been coughing up blood for two or three days. Porter "bled her 12 oz.," applied a blister to her sternum, bathed her feet in warm water, and gave her table salt "as recommended by professor Rush." Yet, Porter did not always feel comfortable in adhering to Rush's methods. For example, he documented his reasons for bleeding Daniel Whitman twenty-four ounces on one January morning and then twelve ounces more that evening. He continued to bleed him up until the following Sunday morning, but more moderately. On January 29, Porter wrote that "should the too cautious practitioner object to the profuse bleeding employed in this case, the following facts will be a most satisfactory reply." He justified his actions by stating that his patient suffered delirium while the pulse remained "full and hard" even after bloodletting. After two more bleedings, the patient's reason returned, and Porter wrote that "whenever sufficient blood was drawn, it operated rather like a charm than an ordinary remedy."[32] The fact that Porter deemed it necessary to defend himself to an imaginary physician who was "too cautious" suggests that he considered profuse bleeding not "an ordinary remedy" or practice in Massachusetts. Perhaps he felt compelled to vindicate his "Rush-like" treatment of Whitman to himself because, as my survey of the practice of five of Porter's peers demonstrates, Massachusetts physicians seldom turned to aggressive bloodletting as a treatment.[33]

As another mainstay in the heroic therapeutic arsenal, calomel (or mercurous chloride) was purportedly a widely prescribed mercurial drug that acted as a strong cathartic. The physicians at MGH who practiced expectant medicine did at times prescribe calomel: "records of actual practice (in hospitals) show that throughout the antebellum period, the regular physicians most vocal in their allegiance to the healing power of nature, including some who openly professed their therapeutic skepticism, still prescribed active treatments, including most of the mainstays of the orthodox material medica."[34] Calomel was not abruptly rejected, though its use steadily declined. The percentage of patients for whom doctors prescribed mercurial drugs dropped by 51 percent in the 1830s, to 41 percent in the 1840s, and 29 percent in the 1850s.[35]

My own research shows that private practice physicians seemed more restrained in their use of mercurial preparations. The three doctors practicing before 1793—Mosman, Lowe, and William Williams—prescribed mercurial drugs modestly: while Mosman showed no use of mercurial remedies, Lowe used them 5 percent of the time, and Williams 4 percent (see table 1.9). Yet, even those practicing at the supposed height of heroic intervention, Mosman and William Williams, did not use calomel or other mercurial drugs frequently (1% for Mosman and 4% for William Williams). In the 1820s, as the use of mercurial drugs—especially calomel—was receiving public criticism, Williams increased his use slightly from 4 percent to 6. Risk-averse Snow prescribed mercurial compounds 4 percent of the time. Stephen Williams exhibited the highest use of calomel, at 7 percent in the late 1830s.

The explanation for the low use of calomel and other mercurial drugs throughout the period may be found by reviewing the use of cathartics in general. Cathartics comprised a significant portion of the medicine prescribed in private practice. Mosman increased his use of cathartics slightly (17% from 1786 to 1793; 20–21% from 1802 to 1820), while William Williams increased his use of cathartics significantly (25% from 1786 to 1791 to 33% from 1804 to 1806; see table 1.9) during the first decades of the nineteenth century when heroic therapeutics were common. The physicians who practiced during the hailstorm of criticism of heroic therapeutics—Snow, William Williams, and Stephen Williams—all continued to employ cathartics as a mainstay of their practices (14%, 36%, and 24%, respectively). Thus, the cachet of calomel and other mercurial remedies may not have been drawn on for treatment frequently, but doctors heavily utilized cathartics in general. Snow, who practiced expectant medicine, showed the lowest percent of cathartic use (14%), as one would expect. But even among those who employed cathartics at the highest percentages—William Williams and Lowe (36% and 25%, respectively)—the types of cathartics they prescribed were more likely to be mild-to-moderate rather than violent- or strong-acting kinds (see table 1.10).[36] This body of evidence demonstrates that private practitioners in Massachusetts prescribed mercurial drugs less often than they did milder types of cathartics. This was true in all the periods under consideration.

The wide usage of cathartics by all five practitioners across the entire fifty-year span may indicate the prevalence of constipation and other gastrointestinal disturbances in patients. Problems with digestion remained a central concern for patients throughout the eighteenth and nineteenth centuries. In 1756 John Hartshorn recorded: "Went to See Mrs. Liscow complained of Pain in her Intestines which gave her flushes of heat, I found She had been costive for 3 or 4 days."[37] He gave her a cathartic that resulted in many bowel movements and relief from her intestinal pain. Hartshorn frequently treated patients whose constipation—like Liscow's—had lasted for long periods.[38]

A significant portion of prescriptive literature dedicated to changes in diet to prevent illnesses (including digestive ailments such as constipation) testifies to the prevalence of diagnosed gastrointestinal problems. Thomas A. Horrocks found that 16 percent of the 1,785 almanacs between 1646 and 1861 that he examined provided regimen advice for preserving health. That figure rose to 25 percent in the second half of the eighteenth century. As Horrocks's data suggest, the relationship of diet to digestion was not a new concept. Yet in the first three decades of the nineteenth century that relationship became seminal to health advocates, beginning with the influence of a Parisian physician, François Broussais (1772–1838), who argued that almost every disease stemmed from gastrointestinal problems.[39] Warner documents the Parisian influence on Boston physicians, which suggests that Boston physicians would have been inclined to focus on gastrointestinal ailments.[40]

Stephen Williams claimed that among his own patients the most common complaints were coughs, fevers, and bowel disturbances.[41] A perusal of mid-nineteenth-century patients' diaries and physicians' casebooks attests to the validity of Williams's claim. George Chandler's casebook documents that Mr. Forbush had suffered from "costiveness" for several years, taking cathartics on and off.[42] One of Dr. Sargent's patients said that he himself had "never been 'in [the] hands of a Dr.' in his life," but on November 19, 1840, he sought Sargent's help due to the pain of costiveness and hemorrhoids.[43]

New Englanders' diets contributed to part of the endemic digestive problems, for they changed over time in ways that ensured constipation.[44] Contemporary critics, especially those advocating vegetarianism, admonished Americans for the enormous amount of meat and starch they ate while ignoring fresh fruits and vegetables. This diet made "constipation the national curse of the first four or five decades of the nineteenth century." Most families' meat intake included salt pork and beef, with vegetables often used merely as a base for sauces accompanying their meats. By the mid-nineteenth century potatoes and cabbage became the main vegetables served as a side dish. Popular health journals complained of Americans' penchant for salty meat and few vegetables, often connecting their diets to struggles with constipation. In 1860, the *Ladies' Home Magazine* quoted *Hall's Journal of Health* advice that readers should eat apples, for they often relieved constipation.[45] Thus, an apple a day would keep the doctor away.

Diets often differed among the various classes, of course. For example, members of the urban "upper crust" could afford wheat flour for lighter breads rather than the coarse grains used for breads eaten by the working classes. Apple cider had replaced beer as the fermented drink of choice by the mid-eighteenth century.[46] Prior to 1850, cider, rum, and whiskey were the alcoholic beverages of choice. Although the temperance movement arose among the middle class, eventually attacking the ingestion of cider and beer, many drank cider daily. Coffee replaced tea as the nonalcoholic drink of choice; Americans drank it almost four times as much as tea.[47] Diets that consisted of fatty, salty meats with light breads and fermented or caffeinated drinks created dehydrated bodies with little fiber, a formula for constipation. The frequency of constipation documented in medical records arose as a result of both the physicians' focus on gastrointestinal problems and the change in New Englanders' diets. Thus, it is little wonder that cathartics (usually of mild-to-moderate action) became a mainstay of medical practice.

Alongside bleeding and calomel, emetics, or "pukes," provided the most inspiration for caricatures of orthodox medicine. Given their association with orthodox medicine, emetics were handed out by the physicians in this study surprisingly seldom, especially in comparison to Warner's findings. At the MGH, the physicians prescribed emetics 22 percent of the time in the 1830s, 12.1 percent in the 1840s, and 7 percent in the 1850s, a steady decrease. However, private physicians never dispensed emetics more than 6 percent of the time. In the eighteenth century, before heroic therapeutics supposedly dominated, Mosman, Lowe, and Williams prescribed emetics in moderate amounts, 3 to 5 percent (see table 1.9). During the heroic era, Mosman increased his use from 3 to 5 percent. William Williams appeared unimpressed by heroic therapeutics; he changed his puking very little during the 1800s, rising to 6 percent in the 1820s. Snow predictably used emetics in 2 percent of his treatments, while Stephen Williams employed them less than 1 percent of the time.[48]

Emetics would have produced a discernible reaction, but perhaps one that was not well tolerated by patients.[49] For example, patients with lung problems were treated with emetics to combat an accumulation of phlegm. On October 7, 1833, Deborah Fiske wrote to her husband that she was in considerable pain and that "Dr. Warren came & said it was owing to the accumulation of phlegm & that an emetic would relieve me. I took one immediately, it operated well & I have since been better."[50] However, emetics, especially when taken numerous times, often resulted in painful sore throats.

To offset the harsh side effects of emetics, doctors prescribed opiates for pain relief. Justin Colley awakened on April 27, 1810, with violent pains in his stomach. Jacob Porter prescribed opium and a repeated dose of an emetic and cathartic. When these medications did not work, he gave Colley "emetic wine" in small doses until he began to vomit. Porter recorded that the vomiting "left him dull and drowsy but free of pain."[51] Opiates helped patients tolerate emetics.

The limited use of emetics may be explained by the physician's perception of having little control over the operation of the drugs, their fear of side effects, or patients' refusal to ingest them. The differences between hospital and private-practice use of emetics may be explained by the differing medical experiences of patient populations. After all, the patients in the MGH wards tended to be working-class and often nonpaying; consequently, they were not in a position to dictate their therapy. Patients in private practice, who paid their physicians, had more influence over their bodies. They could negotiate with doctors over treatment, or reduce the dosage, or discontinue taking their medicine entirely, which shows how patients influenced therapeutic approaches.

Many Massachusetts patients consulted with physicians for pain management. Historian Edward Shorter contends that "patients sought treatment or took time off for relatively few of their symptoms" until after the 1820s, when "a major part of the patient's story will be the expansion of the symptom pyramid to include lesser and lesser complaints." He questions whether the "traditional patient" was less "sensitive to pain and discomfort than we are, or just more stoical about them."[52] The prescribing trends for opiates among the five physicians in my sample, however, challenge Shorter's general argument. Physicians prescribed opiates and narcotics frequently throughout late eighteenth century and well into the nineteenth century. William Williams, the least likely to prescribe opiates, had increased his use of them from 11 to 13 percent by the 1820s. Mosman increased his prescriptions of opiates as well, from 12 percent in the late eighteenth century to 20 percent in the early nineteenth century (see table 1.9). By the 1830s, Stephen Williams became the highest prescriber of opiates—as much as 25 percent. Warner's data demonstrate that the increased use of opiates continued. MGH practitioners' use of opiates increased from 45 percent in the 1830s to 54 percent in the 1840s, and up to 63 percent in the 1850s.[53]

Overall, with the exception of Williams, the doctors showed a steady increase in the use of opiates by about the same percentages as their use of cathartics. Pain relief was a major component of medical practice throughout the period.[54] Thus, data suggest that patients were not more stoical about pain in the eighteenth century. Even before the 1800s, when the use of pain medications began to increase steadily, pain management had always been an important aspect of medical care.

Certainly, patients had access to opiates so that they might medicate themselves.[55] In fact, the medicine chests sold in Boston by Dr. A. Seaton included paregoric elixir and camphor, two of the most widely prescribed narcotic mixtures.[56] However, many patients feared overdosing during self-administration. Doctors needed to be consulted in the use of narcotics because they had more experience with all sizes and ages of patients than nonpractitioners did. In *Domestic Medicine* (1769), Buchan cautioned readers against overdosing with opium. Under the section titled "On Poisons" he wrote: "Opium, being frequently taken by mistake, merits particular attention. It is indeed a valuable medicine when taken in its proper quantity, but as an overdose proves a strong poison."[57] Around 1850, John Ware lectured to his medical students at Harvard that "the knowledge of the proper administration of opiates makes more difference in physicians than any other one thing."[58] Both Buchan's and Ware's awareness of patients' demands for good advice in pain management signifies the centrality of that advice to a successful medical practice.

George Chandler wrote a diatribe on the subject of the mishandling of opium and quinine at home. On January 10, 1839, he recorded in his casebook how one widow who suffered poor health was constantly undermined by "her perversity of disposition & neglect of even an approach to decent attention in the Boors who croaked & prowled about her." He feared that several factors—"the family jars [of medicine]," her "cruel disease," and the poverty of the house whereby the "powers of winter blasts on her almost naked person, [and] the murky damps of a pestiferous cell"—would kill her.[59] Chandler expressed disgust at the negligence of the women's care by the boorish family members prior to his attendance; they frequently mishandled her medications or ignored her. Opium could bring relief from pain if properly administered; or it could bring death in the hands of neglectful or ignorant caregivers. A doctor of Chandler's experience could oversee its proper use.

Throughout the period studied, opiates brought relief to patients for many ailments. For example, doctors often prescribed opiates and other types of sedatives for convulsive fits. Porter gave laudanum to a nine-month-old girl who suffered from long bouts of crying and fits of convulsions that lasted eight to ten minutes.[60] Her mother was instructed to "give laudanum at the commencement of every periodical return [of the convulsions] and as her feet were frequently cold to bathe them, whenever that was the case in warm water."[61] Opiates sedated patients to prevent physical harm due to convulsions, thus providing relief to them, their families, and their caretakers.

As mentioned earlier, opiates were often dispensed in tandem with cathartics and emetics. Sargent treated Bridget, an Irish immigrant servant girl, for "eruptions of large white blotches on face and neck" that spread to the rest of her body and turned red. Given ipecac and jalap, Bridget later complained of pains in her throat and abdomen and was given opium tincture with cinnamon and cream of tartar for pain relief.[62]

Narcotics were not just ingested but applied topically for relief of pain as well. Sargent administered opiate drops as an eye treatment. Given that protective goggles were not in common use in the workplace, whether farm or factory, Sargent and other physicians treated many eye injuries.[63] Mrs. Lucretia Bertody came to Sargent with a painful right eye intolerant to light. Sargent wrote that he "diluted laudanum" that "was applied to eye" and he "found [her to be] very grateful."[64]

Physicians frequently used morphine and opium postoperatively as well. Caroline Barrett White recorded in her diary the harrowing experience of witnessing her sister undergoing surgery to remove a tumor in the right breast. The surgery was performed in their home while family assisted:

> Drs. Hitchcock and Page of Fitchburg arrived—at sight of whom we *all* trembled with anxious fears. . . . They proceeded at once to get her in bed, & position—and as soon as she could calm herself a little—commenced *etherization*—I never saw any one inhale ether before—and had no idea it was so painful to witness—When they had her well under its influence & were ready to begin the removal of the tumor, they gave me the ether to administer as required for complete unconsciousness. While G. Martin held her right arm in position so they could work handily. So we were both obliged to witness the bloody operation which lasted an *hour*. The wound or incision was about five inches in length and after the removal of the whole breast—it was sewed up & kept in place by plasters—It was terrible to me. . . . The return of consciousness was the most agonizing to poor L. . . . She suffered intolerably for an hour or two—but after the Dr. administered a morphine powder, the pain gradually subsided.[65]

White's passage on her sister's mastectomy reminds us that medical care was observed and on display in the home. In many cases, there was no separation of clinical practice from domesticity, and a loved one's comfort through pain management would be paramount to family observers.

The increase in the use of opiates can be partially explained by the "more self-conscious emphasis on palliation" in terminal cases in the nineteenth century.[66] Daniel Child noted on September 5, 1846, that his brother Samuel "continues very unwell." By September 15, he wrote that "Brother Samuel [was] failing gradually, and thought, by his physician to be very near the end." The family congregated at the father's home, where Samuel was found to be "still alive and quiet under the effects of opiates." By 10:00 p.m. that night Samuel had died, never having awakened from his opium-induced sleep.[67]

Warner documents a notable development among doctors practicing expectant medicine in the 1840s—the "self-conscious emphasis on palliation" whereby the physician "could create a healing environment enhanced by the alleviation of pain in which the natural healing processes could proceed." The use of opiates for palliative care occurred in private practice as well as hospital wards. In terminal cases, patients expected relief from suffering rather than the "active cure of disease."[68]

Given the variety of uses of opiates and the prevalence of pain, it is not surprising that opiates and sedatives comprised a goodly portion of medical remedies in private practice. Oddly, two contradictory theories existed regarding the effect of opium on the body. On the one hand, John Brown—fellow student and inspiration to Rush—believed that opium was a stimulant needed to treat a large list of "debilitating diseases" such as gout and chronic rheumatism. On the other hand, many physicians believed that opium acted as a sedative that aided in the treatment of a range of diseases such as convulsions, spasmodic pain, and putrid sore throats. Thus, these "opposing medical concepts cohabited within the therapeutics field"; the addition of Brown's theory, "which viewed illnesses as being due to a lack of stimulation, contributed to the increased use of opium."[69] Competing theories of how opium affected the body meant that physicians in both therapeutic camps could justify their prescriptions for opium.

Patients' access to opiates increased owing to a profusion of drug advertisements. Daily newspapers multiplied from twenty in 1800 to four hundred by 1860, and as historian James Young states, "the nostrum promoter counted on the press as the most likely vehicle to carry his message to potential customers."[70] As daily papers flourished so did the number of proprietary brands of drugs. For example, in 1771 a Philadelphia drug catalog had listed no American brands, whereas by 1804 a New York catalog showcased eighty to ninety nostrums, the majority of which were American-made. Add the number of European brands still advertised and sold in America and the availability of prepared remedies can be seen to have increased markedly.[71] Many of the advertised prepared remedies had opium as an ingredient, such as the widely prescribed Dover's Powder. Nostrum promoters increased their sales through product recognition. Nostrum makers could sell their products directly to patients. Thus it is not hard to imagine that patients might demand that physicians use products familiar to them, especially if those patients had enjoyed previous success with certain remedies.

Where the five physicians showed the greatest variation was in whether on most visits they gave their patients any medicine at all.[72] To measure this, I looked for ledger entries showing that the doctor charged for "visit and advice" rather than listing medicines or designating "visit and sundry meds." For the period before 1800, in these practices the existing data reveal that physicians almost invariably gave their patients medicines if they visited. Mosman and Lowe visited without dispensing medicines less than 1 percent of the time. There was no change for Mosman in his later practice

(1802–20). William Williams did not prescribe medicine 7 percent of the time between 1786 and 1791; this decreased to 3 percent between 1804 and 1806 and rose back up to 7 percent in the 1820s. Snow (practicing between 1827 and 1828) represents the practitioner with the highest percentage of visiting without medicating—38 percent. Stephen Williams comes in second with 9 percent (see table 1.9).

Stephen Williams championed the concept of self-limiting diseases and the expectant method of medical practice espoused by Jacob Bigelow and others in Boston. For Williams, the physician's role was to assist nature in her work. Nature would cure the patient, and the physician's assistance should take the form of a "mild internal practice." However, he also admitted that "we [have] given less medicine than formerly, but whenever we do give it, we administer it in as heroic doses as ever."[73] His prescribing patterns appear to bear this out. Although he was the second most likely to visit without prescribing a medicine (9%), Williams used calomel the most (7%), employed strong cathartics (9%, tied for most frequent user with his father; see table 1.10), and was the most likely to prescribe opiates.

Snow's prescribing habits indicate a doctor who practiced what he preached. He prescribed no medicine 38 percent of the time, he bled less than 1 percent, and was the lowest to prescribe cathartics (14%) and second lowest to prescribe emetics (2%). Of those practicing after 1820, Snow demonstrated a commitment to dispensing no medicine, attesting to his belief in helping nature to restore health rather than intervening. William Williams and his son Stephen certainly gave medicines more frequently than Mosman and Lowe had earlier, but they may have not been able to desist from handing out medicines to the same extent as Snow. The difference rests in the culture in which they practiced medicine, Boston compared to Deerfield.

Like many cities in the country, Boston experienced a specialization of labor during the nineteenth century. Just as factories began to separate labor into more and more distinct tasks until the work was divided into many subspecialty skills, so did medical practice begin to move toward more specialization.[74] According to Richard Shryock, the trend toward division of labor in urban medical practices began when physicians gradually abandoned drug selling during the period from 1790 to 1820.[75] Snow's practice, and other Boston physicians' account books, indicate that this shift began with medical practices in Boston before it occurred in western

Massachusetts. The separation of tasks—medical consultation from the dispensing of remedies—in the urban medical practice meant records noting "visit and prescription" or simply "visit and advice," together with charges, sufficed.

Snow's practice differed from that of Stephen Williams's Deerfield practice in other ways as well. Snow forged a professional identity within an important medical center. Acquisition of experience in institutions such as a hospital or an almshouse was less frequent in the United States than in Europe. Boston, however, housed a prominent medical school, Harvard, as well as several institutions offering physicians and medical students a chance to gain medical experience—the almshouse, the Boston Dispensary, Massachusetts General Hospital, and the Asylum for Indigent Boys and Female Orphanage Asylum, to name a few.[76] Snow was one of the directors of the Penitent Females' Refuge, which provided him with both medical experience and a reputation for benevolence.[77] Thus, Snow obtained experience at the domestic bedside and with the natural history of a disease which could be found in a clinic, in hospital wards and autopsy rooms.[78] In addition, Snow could easily attend medical lectures and Massachusetts Medical Society meetings, sharing professional solidarity with the most vocal proponents of expectant medicine—Jacob Bigelow and James Jackson. He wrote and sold a religious schoolbook, *Dr. Snow's First Principles of English Spelling and Reading*, which was frequently advertised in the *Boston Recorder and Religious Telegraph*, providing proof to readers (who might be potential patients) of his good and pious character.[79] All these activities required little travel on Snow's part and added much to his professional reputation.

A good professional reputation was an important step toward a successful medical career. Warner argues that an individual physician's status "came more from his own interactions with patients and other practitioners and from such factors as family and community connections."[80] Hence, Snow's regular attendance at medical society meetings, his connection to religious organizations such as the Massachusetts Sabbath School Union, his election to the school committee in 1824, and his directorship of a charitable refuge for women—all played a large part in his success.[81] Yet, a doctor could not sustain a practice of medicine unless enough patients were convinced, or at least could be persuaded, of the merits of his approach to medicine. Snow's expectant method would have found a welcoming audience among middle-class Bostonians (as will be discussed later). Snow parlayed his experience, benevolent activities, and medical approach into a successful practice.

The professional landscape in Stephen Williams's rural New England practice was very different. The bulk of his practice involved the "here-and-now focus on livelihood, neighbors, and practical care." Stephen Stowe argues in regard to country practices in the South that rural doctors had to struggle with the tension between two desires. One involved the attachment to their professional training in an intellectual realm; the other was the more practical concern of belonging to the everydayness of the community.[82] Or to put it another way, the country doctor sometimes experienced a tension between his role as a healer to his patients, along with their expectations, and his identity as a scientist.[83]

Williams serves as a good example of these conflicting desires. His obituary in *Boston Medical and Surgical Journal* (1855) makes it clear that he had aggressively sought to create his professional identity through scholarly pursuits. He became a member of the State Medical Society of Vermont in 1815 and the Massachusetts Medical Society in 1817.[84] He lectured on medical jurisprudence whenever his practice would allow, at Berkshire Medical Institute (1823), the College of Physicians and Surgeons, New York (1838), and Dartmouth College (1838). Yet, it was a struggle to participate in these professional activities. When he went to lecture in New York in 1838, he had to hire Darwin Hamilton to take over his practice for eighteen days. A year later, Williams noted that he had to borrow twenty-five dollars from Luther B. Lincoln "for my western tour" to Willoughby University in Ohio to lecture.[85] In other words, Williams had to balance his involvement in the scholarly world of his profession with the pragmatic need to make a living. This necessity would have included his figuring out a way to adhere to his theoretical beliefs while tending to his patients' demands.

The patients Williams treated came from a variety of socioeconomic situations. To his more educated and religiously liberal patients, giving advice while not necessarily prescribing medications would have been acceptable. To those patients with less knowledge of—or less faith in—the "new concepts" in medicine, a physician who did not "do" something would not be acceptable. Evidence of the concern over balancing science with patients' wishes can be seen in Worthington Hooker's pamphlet "*Dissertation on the Respect Due the Medical Profession, and the Reasons That It Is Not Awarded by the Community* (1844). Hooker described physicians becoming more interested in "patient-getting" than in "patient-curing." In other words, he decried physicians who were more interested in attracting patients by catering to their whims than in practicing good medicine. He made the distinction between urban and rural medicine: "The evil of which we speak [patient-getting] exists to a greater extent in the country than in large towns and cities." He attributed this to the fact that towns had sufficient numbers of physicians to form professional medical communities.[86] Both Snow and Williams understood that practicing good medicine meant that physicians assist nature, allowing nature to heal some diseases. But neither were they therapeutic nihilists; they dispensed medicines when they deemed them necessary. Yet Snow adhered to the theory of self-limiting diseases more faithfully than Stephen Williams, perhaps due to his greater commitment to the expectant approach but more likely because they practiced in two different medical communities.

Whether a physician prescribed medicines or not, and what kind, depended on patients' expectations. In hospitals, medical theory prevailed; patients' therapeutic demands could remain unmet due to the "degree of physician control over therapy that was common in hospitals but difficult to exercise in private practice."[87] This can be seen when Dr. Fisher called on Mary Louisa Child in February 20, 1846. Daniel Child wrote: "Mary Louisa yet remains unwell. Doct. Fisher prescribes but little for her, thinking some disease may be about to develop itself by a cutaneous eruption." Mrs. Child was relieved when the next day Fisher "called at one o'clock and prescribed *active* [her emphasis] medicine for Mary Louisa."[88] Fisher may have felt compelled to prescribe medicine in response to Mrs. Child's anxiety. As an attending physician at Massachusetts General Hospital,[89] he could have refused to bleed a patient or give patients calomel while servicing the wards, but when treating the Child family as part of his private practice, he could not exert as much control.

Hooker's writings further illustrate the pressure to please patients. He bemoaned the dishonest way in which some physicians were overcoming patients' fears over the use of strong cathartics, such as calomel. Many doctors circumvented their patients' objections to calomel by combining calomel with another substance and telling them to take the "quieting powder." Hooker described how the ruse was accomplished: "Armenian bole, as it is an inert substance and yet has a decided color, is quite a favorite article with those who practice this concealment, and many a physician has gained much credit from the wonderful effects of his pink powders, his patient not once dreaming that they are calomel in disguise." Hooker did not suggest that patients should always be told everything for their own good, but objected to doctors giving in to patients' demands rather than practicing honest medicine.[90]

Due to the pervasiveness of costiveness and other intestinal problems, cathartics were a major component of doctors' treatments. As such, some patients negotiated for mild cathartics, avoiding strong cathartics like calomel. Dr. Jacob Porter's interactions with Melinda Ford give us a glimpse of possible negotiations over treatment of stomach pains. The doctor had prescribed a nonmercury cathartic that had worked eight to nine times the day before. Ford was comfortable during the day, but a very acute pain returned. On December 22, 1809, Porter wrote that Ford discontinued her use of the nitric acid he prescribed. She complained that the cathartic "brought on a sickness at the stomach." Porter encouraged her to continue to take it. "I remarked that if the disorder was not removed in 2 or 3 days, under these remedies, it would be necessary to calomelise her and endeavored by several arguments to unlock her mercurial fears," he recorded.[91]

Porter's transformation of calomel into an action verb—"calomelises"— hints at the power of the drug. The strong and painful intestinal contractions brought on by the ingestion of calomel understandably inspired "mercurial fears" in many patients. Yet, Porter understood that severe constipation could become dangerous and required strong treatments. As data show, an abundance of cathartics existed for the initial treatment of constipation without having to resort to strong cathartics such as calomel, thus circumventing any need to overcome patients' fears or resistance.

Physicians acquiesced to patients' demands over other treatments as well. Patients in pain often received opiates. Yet when they were taken too frequently constipation became a common side effect. In the eighteenth century, apprentice John Hartshorn yielded to a patient's wishes: "Went to See Bourke, he got some Ease by his Last night's anodyne, I gave him another tonight, tho' it was bad Practice but he wou'd not consent to purging."[92] Presumably, Hartshorn believed that a cathartic for purging would have relieved the stomach problem but instead prescribed anodyne, a narcotic, to mask the pain, even though he considered it to be bad medical practice.

Nineteenth-century physician Joseph Sargent found himself in a similar predicament. He attempted to dissuade one of his patients from taking any more opium because she had had one "gathering" (bowel movement) in many days. Sargent suggested an application of leeches for inflammation of the hip and external narcotics for the pain. He was informed by the patient's husband that she "did not make the application above Right Ilium [right hip] that I directed—having a horror of leeches." The husband wrote a letter to Sargent stating that she "has taken no opium until 4 or 5 days ago ... of late she has suffered exceedingly from pain in her face & neck shifting at times to her side & hip & bowels which has considerably reduced her strength."[93] At this point, the patient began taking opium again. Sargent advised her once again not to take it, but his negotiations with the patient appear to have been unsuccessful.

Of course, some patients exercised their agency by simply not taking the medicine their physician prescribed. One of Dr. George Chandler's patients suffered from chronic constipation. When the condition worsened, the patient came to Chandler, who pronounced that the problem arose "from neglecting to take medicine [cathartics the patient was prescribed earlier] when costive."[94] Jacob Porter faced similar noncompliance on the part of some of his patients. For example, he documented a patient who refused the blisters he "twice advised" be applied to her breast. Another patient regretted his noncompliance with Porter's instructions: "I do not doubt, says he, but that if I had taken the drops regularly, as you ordered me, my face would have been perfectly well."[95] Patients' expectations and compliance or noncompliance dictated therapeutic trends as much as medical theories.

As Mosman's, Lowe's, and Williams's practices substantiate, the use of purges and pukes predated Rush's rise to fame in the aftermath of the 1793 yellow fever epidemic.[96] The prescribing patterns of Mosman, Lowe, William Williams, Snow, and Stephen Williams from the 1780s to the 1830s further demonstrate that Massachusetts physicians did not habitually use calomel or any other mercurial drugs, despite charges made by nostrum advertisers that regular physicians overused them. Nor, apparently, did they bleed as copiously or as frequently as claimed by contemporary medical sects and later historians. Physicians' prescribing patterns in private practice suggest a revised understanding of the criticisms that emerged by the mid-nineteenth century as not in fact due to a prolonged patient dissatisfaction with heroic therapies.

Heroic depletive therapy was never employed as brutally as it has been depicted. As one historian of medicine explains: "Historians' image of such practice as typical results largely from a reliance on retrospective evidence, the recollections of physicians in the middle or late nineteenth century about how bad practice had been in earlier years. Such stories must be read for what they were, namely, self-satisfied statements about how much medicine had improved."[97] Dramatic incidences such as nineteenth-century accounts of George Washington being bled to death, linger in historical memory, coloring our understanding of American medicine. Regional hospital studies demonstrate that Massachusetts physicians did not practice heroic medicine as aggressively as their counterparts in hospitals as other regions of the country. This proves to be true in private practice as well.

Analysis here shows that Massachusetts private practitioners had always been moderate in their therapeutic approach before, during, and after Rush's rise to prominence. The doctors often prescribed mild laxatives and opiates, demonstrating that in the case of two widely documented medical complaints in patients' diaries—constipation and pain—patients' expectations were met. Also, when employed, "heroic medicines were not just harsh, they were flexible and varied and subjective."[98] The variations lay in the medical culture (shaped by patient expectations) in which each of these physicians practiced. What has colored historians' understanding of private practice in early America are the numerous depictions of orthodox practitioners that were based more on caricatures of Rush and his theories rather than on how patients and physicians negotiated therapeutics in actual private practice.[99] In fact, this is a narrative of continuity rather than a rise and fall of heroic depletive therapy. Only when patient expectations changed by the mid-nineteenth century did they seek alternative therapies to meet them.

2
Self-Medication in the Nineteenth Century

In the Early Republic, physicians did not enjoy complete authority in matters of illness. Patients could and did treat themselves with home or patent medicines. They sought guidance from family, neighbors, clergymen, and orthodox and unorthodox healers, often mixing a physician's prescription with any advice they had received. Whereas there are numerous daybooks that document physicians' prescribing patterns, to discover the self-medication practices and therapeutic remedies chosen by patients in the late eighteenth to mid-nineteenth century requires scouring through diaries, correspondence, and medical advertisements. Glimpses of self-medicating choices made by transient, impoverished, and working-class patient populations prove even more elusive but can be found in the Massachusetts General Hospital (MGH) intake interviews from the 1820s to the 1850s. Patients chose among many medicinal options, ranging from home remedies to patent medicines to treatments dispensed by a variety of practitioners. In making those choices, they shaped therapeutics.

Patients could either mix their own remedies or buy packaged ones. In fact, many of the packaged compounds dispensed by physicians were directly available to and often self-administered by patients or their families. Lay people who compounded their own medicines could appeal to neighbors and family for help or peruse family cookbooks for recipes. Recipes for home remedies could be found in books such as William Buchan's *Domestic Medicine* (1816) and Lewis Merlin's *The Treasure of Health* (1819). Self-treatment became so popular that the New Haven, Connecticut, publishers of the 1816 edition of *Domestic Medicine* retitled it *Every Man His Own Physician* and added recipes ranging from a cure for jaundice to ketchup that would keep for twenty years.[1] As part of a long tradition, Merlin's *Treasure of Health* provided a collection of recipes purported to cure all kinds of diseases. Many of these recipes dated from two hundred years past.[2]

In the pages of family cookbooks, recipes for green-pea soup as well as plasters for pain relief were printed side by side. Some remedies served both nutritional and medicinal purposes, blurring the distinction between the two. For example, in the eighteenth century newly laid eggs were served to mothers as food and applied externally after birth, "first having been stirred over hot embers in an earthen pipkin, then plastered on a dressing."[3] The tradition of using domestic recipes for medical treatment continued into the nineteenth century. In an 1842 letter, a woman whose uncle and aunt had "both laughed heartily at her prescription for their rheumatism, *Mustard poultices*," stated that "neither of them have it bad enough to resort to such remedies." "It would indeed be worse than the disease," they concluded.[4] An unmarried mason in Boston reported to the house physician at MGH that he often treated his constipation by drinking boiled milk sweetened "with white paper cut up and boiled with it."[5] Indeed, home remedies continue to be used today.

Even superstitious remedies persisted into the nineteenth century. On September 20, 1843, Mary Gardiner Lowell recorded an anecdote told by Dr. Warren demonstrating the "remarkably strong manner [of] the effects of imagination." A woman came to him for treatment of a tumor on her neck. When Warren recommended that the growth be surgically removed, she felt "a great want of resolution to endure the knife, begged him to at least try first some other remedy." He prescribed her an innocuous wash and told her come back. After a fortnight, she returned, her tumor unchanged. She then told the doctor that she had heard of a remedy she would like to try, if he had no objection. She had heard that the touch of a dead man's finger three times on her tumor would cure it. Warren had to resist the impulse to laugh; but "He reflected it was better to humor her." Fortuitously for the patient, a neighbor man lay dead, so the opportunity to test her "folk" remedy presented itself. At the end of the fortnight she returned to Dr. Warren, smiling, and showed him that the tumor had entirely disappeared! He had to concur.[6]

If a patient desired a pre-made remedy, then a profusion of "patent" medicines (although frequently referred to as such, they are more accurately termed "proprietary medicines" because few were actually patented) were advertised in newspapers, pamphlets, and broadsides.[7] The earliest American example, appearing in a 1708 issue of the *Boston News-Letter,* was for the English proprietary medicine named Daffy's Elixir Salutis, a cathartic and diuretic panacea.[8] At this early date, American advertisements simply listed the medicines available at the apothecary's. Eight of these imported remedies—"Bateman's Pectoral Drops, Godfrey's Cordial, Turlington's Balsam of Life, Hopper's Female Pills, Anderson's Scots Pills, Dalby's Carminative, Steer's Opodeldoc, and British Oil—were extensively advertised in the American press" by the mid-eighteenth century.[9]

With the advent of American independence, the ability to compound English medicines in America rather than importing them from England became essential, creating local competition between American-made products and English imports. The new republic fostered "a renewed search by American physicians to discover American herbs which could relieve the American sickness of an 'unrepublican dependence' on European medicines."[10] Nineteenth-century proprietors created eye-catching, columns-long newspaper advertisements for packaged remedies. For example, a notice for Dr. Relfe's Botanical Drops in the *Boston Gazette* featured a drawing of the bottle of drops, along with many testimonials of cures from satisfied customers throughout New England. One patient, a Boston lady, was described as suffering from swollen glands for most of her life, but when she took the drops, "to her astonishment, the whole of the glands were reduced to their natural state, and her health perfectly restored!"[11] The inclusion of drawings and personal testimonies made advertisements more engaging and memorable.

Among the working class, one mother of a five-year-old child who was admitted to MGH on June 2, 1848, reported to Dr. R. K. Jones that her child had always been delicate and feeble. For the last year and a half the child had been treated with "a patent medicine 'Indian cholagogue' and was in the daily use of it when [the] present disease commenced." The mother told Jones that other children had used the same medicine and had been similarly affected. Subsequently, Jones had a sample of the medicine tested and "found [it] to contain arsenic as its active ingredient." "Cholagoga" referred to remedies that purged the bilious humor, based on a long tradition of utilizing remedies to create homeostasis among the four humors.[12]

Nor was it unusual for patients to use remedies obtained from other races. The wife of Andrew Ford had burnt her feet with hot water from a tea kettle and "she used various applications, such as Indian poultice, linseed oil and [illegible word] grease, with some efit [sic]" but as, "she being a heavy mom," she was unable to heal herself she called Dr. Porter for aid.[13] Although it is unclear exactly what Mrs. Ford meant by "Indian poultice," by the eighteenth century communication with Native Americans had led to the adoption of many medicinal uses of different local plants.[14] Perhaps Mrs. Ford was referring to such an adopted preparation. Both examples remind us that domestic remedies originated from many sources.

New England diaries and correspondence attest to the frequent use of proprietary medicines by the middle and upper classes as well. For example, James H. Stuart wrote to his mother in 1846 that "Aunt Martha says she knows of no remedy for the piles but Mr. Douglas who was much afflicted with them tried Dr. Jackson's Pile Embrocation. He says that it is rapidly curing him."[15] Stuart offered to procure a bottle and send it to her. Such remedies were unregulated and available to any purchaser at the apothecary or general store. Newspapers and pamphlets frequently listed where such preparations could be bought directly by the public.

Medical advertisements became so ubiquitous that Dr. Worthington Hooker complained at the annual meeting of the Connecticut Medical Society on May 8, 1844, that the quantity of quack advertisements (as Hooker described them) in the papers of the day "indicate[s] the enormous appetite of the people for empiricism." In one twenty-column paper he counted *eleven* filled with such advertisements. He groused that there were "new medicines constantly appearing in rapid succession, and going quickly through their several stages of rise, acme, and decline" and bemoaned the traitors from "our own ranks" who had deserted the practice of medicine in the hope of attaining a fortune in nostrum making rather than remaining with the "poorly-compensated but noble duties of the true votary of medical science."[16]

Patients could also purchase medicine chests that combined a health guide with prepackaged remedies. Ambrose Seaton advertised his medicinal kit in newspapers. "The Self-Physician, or newly invented Medicine Chest, for family, sea, and plantation use" included bottles labeled and numbered along with a guide describing each ingredient. Seaton also provided instructions on how to treat common ailments such as diarrhea: "give a dose of No. 2 [castor oil], to endeavor to work it off, if it continues, give a vomit of No. 32 [Hippo, an emetic], and a dose of No. 4 [laudanum, an opiate] at bedtime." Seaton also advised patients' families about how to treat common injuries. On the topic of broken bones, he instructed that the limb must be extended. Then "place the ends of the bones as aptly as you can together; apply your splints made of either paste boards, or thin pieces of wood covered with a bit of rag." After guiding the reader through the steps necessary to make a splint, Seaton's instructions suggested that bandages be moistened with No. 27 (which the index revealed as Goulard's or lead extract), "an excellent medicine used externally, for all kinds of injuries." When it came to brain injuries, Seaton prudently advised that they were "generally too serious to be meddled with, but by professional men."[17]

Medically oriented pamphlets and broadsides were even more expansive than newspaper advertisements, including long lists of testimonials from consumers and practitioners. Like newspaper advertisements, pamphlets such as Dr. Gordak's Jelly of Pomegranate and Peruvian Pills, "prepared from mild and innocent vegetables," promised a cure for an array of ailments.[18] The "celebrated and genuine" jelly touted the ability to cure everything from minor ailments such as "Flatulency or Wind" to common conditions such as "Nervous Headache" and "Dyspepsia or Indigestion" to serious afflictions such as "Leprosy."[19]

A person did not have to take Dr. Gordak's word for it. The advertiser solicited testimonials: "those who have received a cure by my medicines are requested, for the benefit of the public, to send their certificates [testimonies]; I will pay postage." After seven pages on how to identify all the illnesses that the jelly cured, the pamphlet included several pages of "certificates." One purported to be from Eliza A. Kirk of Lowell, Massachusetts: "Dr. Gordak—Sir, you recollect I promised a certificate of your Jelly of Pomegranate and Pulmonary Jelly, if it cured me. This will certify that the above medicines cured me of a Cough of very long standing, which no physician wherever I applied could give me satisfaction."[20] But as was the case with many of the testimonials in Gordak's advertisement, no record was found of an Eliza Kirk in Lowell. In fact, of the forty-four names and addresses listed, approximately one-half (a very liberal estimate) could be matched in any way to vital records, city directory, or the U.S. census.

Nostrum makers used testimonials allegedly supplied to them by famous people as well as humble citizens in order to sell their goods. In the case of Gordak's advertisement, half of his "patients" appeared not to exist. This was often the case with other advertisements as well. Testimonials of people who did exist were purchased for a small price or might be given for free. "Men and women, persuaded they had been cured, were eager to volunteer their thanks. . . . [W]hether or not they were aware of it, [they] were looking for a boost in self-esteem, attention from the neighbors"—what in modern parlance might be described as seeking their fifteen minutes of fame.[21]

Almanacs provided another venue for mass advertisement of medical remedies. William Swain bought six pages in the 1832 *Farmers and Mechanics Almanac* to sell his panacea. Due to the popularity of almanacs among all classes, "all the major patent medicine proprietors, and many with a more modest ranking, got in the almanac game." Nostrum sellers attempted to distinguish their products by presenting them in novel forms of advertisement—"a pamphlet the size of a postage stamp," for example.[22] I even found advertisements disguised as children's stories. *Terrific Fight with Savages: A Reminiscence of Border Life,* published by Dr. Herrick & Brother, chemists in Albany, New York, appears at first glance to be a pamphlet featuring a children's story; only in small print does it disclose that it is a "guide to health, wealth and happiness."[23] The pamphlet does indeed contain a short story (three pages in length) telling of the Wyandot Indians who "crossed the Ohio a few miles above Wheeling and committed great depredations," such as killing "an old man whom they found alone in his cabin" and spreading "terror throughout the neighborhood." The next twenty-four pages, however, are devoted to describing the miraculous properties of Herrick's Kid Strengthening Plasters, which could "cure in five hours, pain and weakness of the breast, side and back." Herrick's Sugar-Coated Pills were hailed as an effective medicine that gained a reputation for "beauty, goodness and certainty in the treatment of disease."

Herrick resorted to flagrant hyperbole; he asserted that the sugar-coated pills had procured the "united acclamation of more than FIVE MILLIONS OF HUMAN BEINGS who have used them." Among the pages of testimonials are those from statesmen (no names) and physicians such as Dr. Norman of North Adams, Massachusetts (he did exist), who reportedly had tried these sugar-coated pills.[24] Obviously, parents who read to their children would have been the target of such sales pitches.

Whether advertised in newspapers, pamphlets, or broadsides, eighteenth- and nineteenth-century packaged remedies promised cures for a laundry list of diseases. In the eighteenth century, physicians seemed reluctant to promise that their ministrations provided cures, perhaps to avoid being associated with the wild claims of "quack" remedies. As many regulars complained, advertisements promising cure for diseases flourished in the nineteenth century and helped to create patient expectations of "cure" as a medical outcome.

Whereas personal diaries and journals give us evidence of self-medication among the upper ranks of society, the intake interviews by house physicians at the MGH provide information on self-medication practices among immigrants, skilled and unskilled laborers, widows, down-on-their-luck artisans and professionals, and transient workers. The most common obstacle to discovering the self-medication practices of MGH patients was whether a patient proved too ill, mentally incapacitated, or unable to speak English fluently enough to articulate his or her medical history. For example, a fifty-five-year-old married Irish laborer who suffered from "Disease of Brain" was recorded as "very stupid—incapable of giving an account of himself."[25] Another example was a thirty-four-year-old Irish woman who had been in this country for ten years and worked as a domestic when she was able but could not give her medical history because of mental instability. She was transferred to McLean Insane Asylum on April 29, 1847.[26] Some patients could not speak English well enough for the house doctor to record their health history. But even English-speaking patients were unlikely to know what medicines they had taken. In all the decades reviewed, many were unable to report their medicinal treatments to the house physician (see appendix A, "Medicine, not specified": 11%, 7%, 14% in the 1820s, 1830s, and 1840s, respectively).[27]

Another challenge to analysis of hospital records arises from how house physicians documented the details of patients and their histories. During this period, no standardized form existed. After 1825, all house physicians did seem to include information such as name, age, occupation, origin of birth, family history, individual history, pulse, appearance of tongue, and frequency of bowel movements, to name a few, usually given in prose form and not necessarily in the same order. Some house physicians, such as Drs. Charles Bertody and Jonathan Dalton, Jr., in 1847, wrote long narratives and, on occasion, quoted patients. Others recorded just the bare necessities as they saw them, like William A. Davis in 1840. Thus, it is impossible to give an exact count of how many patients were under the care of a physician immediately prior to their entrance into MGH. Whenever possible I counted instances in which house physicians clearly stated that the patient was *not* under a physician's care for the illness that brought them to the hospital ward. Statements that indicated self-medication included "was in the habit of taking," "was not under medical treatment," "took medicine without medical advice," or "took medicine."[28]

Most patients did not medicate at all before seeking professional care. The percentage of sampled patients who reported not being under a physician's care and not taking medicine increased from 42 percent in the 1820s to 57 percent in the 1830s to 61 percent in the 1840s (see "No Medicine" in appendix A). Data from the MGH dispute depictions by historians that "even for the urban working class, the hospital was seen as a last resort." On the contrary, the increase in patients entering the MGH who did not medicate prior to admission indicates that some patient populations relied on hospital care as their primary source of treatment for particular illnesses. The MGH had earned a good reputation by the 1830s and held an annual subscription drive to fund free beds for patients who could not afford to pay for care, which provides one reason why working-class people increasingly used the hospital as a first response to illness. After 1830, 40 percent of patients received treatment free of charge. Hence, many patients who could not afford any treatment prior to admittance entered the wards of the hospital for initial care.[29] (The need for free health care among particular groups of working people may be explained by changing economic practices and will be discussed in chapter 3.)

Another explanation for the increase in the number of patients who did not self-medicate before admittance to MGH may rest in the types of illnesses hospitals treated. Fevers, digestive ailments, and respiratory illnesses (some of the most common ailments treated) could easily turn deadly.

Many patients feared that limosis dyspepsia (indigestion), a common diagnosis listed in the patient records, could be dysentery. Enecia cauma (inflammatory fever) could be the more serious affliction, enecia typhus. House physicians treated typhus frequently in the period studied, and with only moderate success. In the 1830s, an epidemic of typhus occurred. From the samples obtained, forty-five new patients were listed as being treated for typhus—twenty-two from August 30 to October 14, 1836, alone. Of the forty-five total patients, twenty-nine were listed as "well" when discharged, eight as "recovered," one given no description, and one as "much relieved." Six patients died (a mortality rate of 13%).[30] When a servant contracted typhus, his/her employer would not risk infecting the entire household. Hospital wards, inadequate as they were by modern standards, might offer better conditions in which to recover than a bed in a drafty garret room with little or no care provided by busy housemates.

Although respectable citizens ordinarily would not have submitted themselves to care in hospital wards, on occasion small shopkeepers and skilled artisans did. They could afford to pay a small amount to receive care as long as their wives or other family members kept working. Those who lived in boardinghouses with few community ties present another scenario. A German-born butcher admitted to MGH in September 1836 provides a good example. He suffered from a fever, vomiting, and headache for a week while travelling from Philadelphia to Boston. Concerned that he might have contracted typhus, he sought care at the hospital as his first line of treatment.[31] Even those with longer residency in the city might seek care from a hospital as a first option, as did a twenty-eight-year-old stableman who went there for initial treatment of pulmonary symptoms. As the house physician recorded that the young man had already suffered from typhus twice and cholera once, the stableman might have thought it prudent to go directly to the hospital.

Indeed, knowing at what point to stop treating oneself and consult a professional proved to be one of the most crucial skills in domestic health care. In 1803 Dr. James Parkinson's *Medical Admonitions to Families, respecting the Preservation of Health, and the Treatment of the Sick* instructed families about when to call a physician. The manual contained a reference table that helped patients to determine "the propriety of taking the task of curing it [the disease] on themselves" or calling for professional assistance. In the case of intermittent fevers, for example, Parkinson wrote that "to attempt to furnish the domestic practitioners, with information sufficient, to enable him to undertake the cure of this fever, would be fruitless." This "dangerous malady" warranted consultation with a physician who possessed "knowledge of the human frame and of the diseases to which it is subject."[32] By the 1820s, financially strapped patients could obtain access to doctors with knowledge of fevers through the hospital ward.

As was discussed in chapter 1, cathartics comprised a majority of the therapeutics prescribed in private practice. Use of cathartics by patients prior to admittance mirrored data from private practice.[33] In all three decades, MGH patients who self-medicated also took cathartics most frequently. In the 1820s, 28 percent of the sampled patients for that decade tried to treat their ailments with cathartics. A large portion did not specify what ingredients they ingested, but of those who did, many took calomel or another mercurial as a strong-acting cathartic, while those who chose a mild-to-moderate-acting ingredient took aloes, myrrh, or salt water. Later decades showed similar results (26% and 23% in the 1830s and 1840s, respectively), although in the same decades castor oil became a popular mild cathartic to ingest.

Admitted patients often self-medicated with cathartics for specific gastrointestinal problems, especially constipation (13%, 14%, and 15% in the 1820s, 1830s, and 1840s, respectively; see appendix B), and hospital doctors treated them for other gastrointestinal disorders. Chronic diarrhea was much more likely to be treated at MGH than constipation, which could be self-medicated with cathartics (and was, as the data on self-medication indicates) or, in cases of prolonged "piles," often treated by private practitioners. Chronic diarrhea, dyspepsia (indigestion), and dysentery comprised the top three stomach problems diagnosed in the hospital wards. Diarrhea and indigestion could be signs of a more serious ailment—dysentery—which required proper diet and rest for recovery, both of which were more likely to be found in a hospital ward than in boardinghouses, servant quarters, or other living arrangements of semiskilled or service workers.[34]

Care for injuries, inflammation, and skin rashes in the form of plasters, poultices, and unguents represented one of the most frequently documented self-administered treatments among MGH patients. In the 1820s, doctors reported patients treating their own wounds less frequently than in the 1830s and 1840s (5% in the 1820s; 10% in the 1830s; and 9% in the 1840s; see appendix A). Seeking treatment for work injuries may have become less common as the industrial age unfolded. Recipe books and domestic medicine manuals provide a plethora of remedies for topical treatments. Plasters were often recommended for common injuries such as burns, cuts, and rashes. Lewis Merlin praised the healing properties of the "divine cloth plaster," known in the United States as "Mahy's Cloth," a concoction of olive oil, sugar of lead (or cerussa acetata, a cooling agent), gold litharge (or red lead), myrrh powder (antiseptic), and yellow wax strained and soaked into linen cloth, for all sorts of sores and ulcers. This plaster had the added benefits of being comprised of common ingredients and possessing a shelf life of ten years. Superficial wounds could easily be dealt with at home. Lydia Maria Child, in her book *The American Frugal Housewife* (1833), recommended strong soft soap, mixed with pulverized chalk until "as thick as batter," then placed in a thin cloth or bag and applied to the wound to prevent lockjaw.[35]

Syphilitic patients used plasters as initial treatment of an outbreak. Sufferers with particularly bad outbreaks in Boston could go to MGH for treatment, unlike their counterparts in Philadelphia or New York. Among venereal diseases, syphilis aroused great prejudices in both popular sentiment and hospital trustees. At MGH, Drs. James Jackson and John Collins Warren displayed an unusual sensitivity toward the disease, advocating treatment there and suggesting a separate ward to appease opponents of their proposal.[36] Yet, among the patients sampled at MGH who had a diagnosis listed, only 1 percent obtained treatment for syphilis, suggesting that most of the cases were treated privately, or not at all (see appendix B).

The MGH files bolster data found on prescribing patterns of narcotics in private medical practice. Many patients sought advice on the use of narcotics, as is discussed in chapter 1. Hospital records show that out of patients who reported taking medicines prior to admittance, 4 percent did so with narcotics (see appendix A) Yet private practitioners also recorded many patients who were prescribed narcotics before admittance. This adds evidence supporting the probability that even though patients had open access to narcotics, they often sought medical advice before ingesting them.

Self-medicating and consulting a professional healer could also occur simultaneously. Due to the influence of such studies as Laurel Ulrich's *A Midwife's Tale*, many scholars have assumed that in general, as in obstetrical situations, a doctor was consulted in emergencies and as a last resort. For example, Edward Shorter states that patients were not very willing to turn to doctors because "medicine was held in such low esteem that traditional patients preferred to dose themselves or to seek out an 'alternative' healer." Only when homemade remedies or drugs from alternative healers had failed, Shorter asserts, would patients consult a regular physician, because "it was he who had the 'truly powerful drugs.'"[37]

Middle-class patient diaries as well as the MGH patient files provide evidence to the contrary. Daniel Child recorded in his diary that Dr. Fisher was called in to treat his child, George. Child wrote that Fisher ordered a "white bread poultice on the chest and an emetic," for he feared that George was showing symptoms of the measles. A few days later, when the measles did not disappear, George was treated with Mrs. Otis Everett, Jr.'s preserved ginger (which acted as a stimulating tonic) and castor oil. George mended rapidly. In this case, the doctor was consulted first, and when professional treatment did not work satisfactorily, Child turned to a neighbor's advice. In another instance, Child took nitric acid given to him by his doctor, but hedged his probability of successful recovery from gravel by eating onions for their medicinal properties, as amateur healer Miss Hovey had advised.[38]

Further evidence can be found among the working class. A person's occupation could predict a need to rely on a hodgepodge of medical treatments. For instance, a twenty-three-year-old married seaman from Cape Cod reported to Jonathan Dalton, house physician at MGH in 1847, that he had "tried [a] vegetable diet for a year at a time, & the prescription of various quacks & regular physicians c̄ [with] some benefit."[39] As a sailor, he would have had difficulty obtaining regular care from one physician and thus treated his dyspepsia with a combination of self-medication, "quack nostrums," and prescriptions from regular practitioners.

Throughout the period studied, physicians, for the most part, seemed tolerant of (or perhaps resigned to) self-remedies and self-medication. In 1809, Jacob Porter treated nine-month-old Loisa Pool with prescribed calomel and jalap. On a follow-up visit, Loisa's mother informed Porter that "she had some pink[root] and senna steeped, which I [Porter] readily consented that they should give at night."[40] Nor was this an isolated case. Porter documents several incidents in which the patient proposed a remedy to which he would "readily consent."[41] After all, Porter could hardly argue against the use of pinkroot or senna, given that he used them in his own practice.

Physicians utilized many prepackaged remedies as well. Some of the most prevalent among the Massachusetts physician account books I studied were Dr. James's Powder (diaphoretic), Dr. Steer's Opodeldoc (panacea liniment), and Dr. Glauber's Salt (cathartic). In his late-eighteenth-century interleaved almanac, Chandler Robbins, a preacher-physician in Plymouth, Massachusetts, noted his use of "patent" medicines. His favorites included Dr. Hill's Pectoral Balsam ("ye best invented Remedy for *Cough, Consumption, Asthmatic*"), Dr. Hill's Elixir of Bardana ("a safe & absolute Cure for y[e] *Rheumatism*), and Dr. Hill's Essence of Water Docks (an "absolute Cure for scurvy, Leprosy and Cutaneous Disorders").[42] A passage recorded in Hugh Hodge's medical ledger (which he appears to have used as commonplace book as well) similarly illustrates that physicians were not necessarily hostile to self-remedies in the nineteenth century. Hodge, under the heading "On the Patient or his Friend suggesting a Remedy to his Physician," paraphrased the writings of John Gregory, an expert on medical ethics, stating that "their proposal may be a good one; it may even suggest to the ablest Physician what perhaps till then might have not have occurred to him." Some physicians might claim that to do so would undermine the "Dignity of the Profession," but Hodge believed this exemplified a mean and selfish view.[43] Many physicians, such as Hodge, viewed healing as a collaborative effort.

Orthodox healers tolerated patients self-medicating but had various reactions to patients who had already sought care from unorthodox physicians.[44] Regular physicians' reactions to such patients were at best noncommittal and at worst contemptuous, depending on the temperament of the practitioner or the nature of the unorthodox treatment. Joseph Sargent did not provide much commentary when he recorded that a Miss McFarland, an eighteen-year-old, treated by him for a "severe dry tight cough," had "lately been taking roots & herbs under an Indian Doctress."[45] Rebecca Packard wrote to her father, the Reverend Asa Packard, that "Mr. Emerson by employing a certain Dr. Hewitt, a quack bone setter, recovered the use of his limb in a few hours and is now perfectly well."[46] It is hard to know how Rebecca perceived Hewitt. She calls him a quack yet pronounces Mr. Emerson healed without any comment. On April 4, 1845, Dr. Henry Barrett, house physician at MGH, wrote that an eighteen-year-old student from Maine had "taken Jone's Pills, a quack nostrum under use of which eruption entirely disappeared leaving him free [from a case of psoriasis] a no. of mos." Although Packard and Barrett used "quack" to describe a medical treatment, both reported a successful outcome. Perhaps to Rebecca and Dr. Barrett the word "quack" was merely a descriptive rather than a derogatory term.[47]

Less tolerant attitudes toward quackery can be found in such communications as those between regular physicians James Jackson, Sr. (attending physician at MGH, 1821–35), and George Shattuck (attending physician at MGH, 1849–55). Mrs. Shattuck recorded in 1840 that Jackson made a morning call and gave the Shattucks an update on the health of an apprentice. "All of us [were] much interested in the illness of a young apprentice, but he had taken a quack now," she wrote, "& will die of course." She stated that the medical profession needed patience in this "age of Charlatanism."[48] Presumably, Mrs. Shattuck's words reflected Drs. Shattuck's and Jackson's lack of tolerance for unorthodox practitioners.

Economic class appears to have determined what type of unorthodox practitioner a patient might consult. Worthington Hooker, MD, had little patience for unorthodox healers, viewing "Homœpathy, Hydropathy, Thomsonism, Eclecticism & c." as "all but upshots of the same radicalism" begun by "crude dreamers."[49] Each, according to Hooker, held a particular appeal for certain categories of patients: he described Thomsonism as a sect that suited those of "the coarser mind," whereas homeopathy (which drew his deepest contempt) attracted "minds which are refined by fashion or education."[50]

Doctors' records and patients' diaries tend to confirm Hooker's claim that homeopathic practitioners attracted more educated people. In the late 1840s James Stuart wrote to his mother about the popularity of homeopathy among their kin: "I hear from Aunt Kate and Carry occasionally, the former has been pretty much sick all winter and is a great advocate of Homeopathy . . . and the same august subject is occupying Uncle William's brain at present."[51] Elizabeth Peabody, in her biography of the famous homeopathic physician William Wesselhoeft, documented his "success in the treatment of scarlet fever [which] opened the hearts of mothers, and forthwith introduced him into the bosom of the most conservative families" of Boston.[52]

As for the working-class patients, of those sampled not one reported using homeopathic medicine. A few patients told their admitting physicians that they had relied on Thomsonian "compositions" for treatment.[53] In 1849, one physician recorded that the patient "has not had treatment except Thomsonian," implying that this was as good as no treatment at all.

A few patients described receiving care from more informal practitioners. A young sailor from Wales had been suffering from severe chest pains intermittently for several months. He had been "under the care of a female who has administered med[icine] for the purpose of 'driving the mercury out of his bones.'" However, Dr. Henry J. Bigelow believed that "his present & past suffering were attributed" to her ministrations. Unfortunately, he did not record the female practitioner's name or the specifics of her treatments.

As in the past, nineteenth-century elderly women in the community served as de facto practitioners of health care. A single, twenty-two-year-old female from East Bridgewater, Massachusetts, who came for treatment at MGH reported that she "was told by an elderly female that she had dropsy," and the elder woman "undertook to cure her of that disease privately & for about 3 months administered various meds: the principal effect" was copious watery discharge with "no relief to dropsy but c [with] sm[all] improvements in other respects."[54]

In the absence of professional advice, patients had to diagnose themselves. This could prove fatal. Mary Gardiner Lowell documented one case showing the unfortunate consequences of self-diagnosis and self-medication that could occur. On March 29, 1844, she referred to an uncle's illness that he himself diagnosed as rheumatism. The family had considered him very ill and encouraged him to seek help. "Not having been so well for some time he came to town to consult Dr. Holmes," Lowell wrote, "and James [Russell] knowing he intended doing so stopped before he went out of town to ask the Doctors opinion when he was extremely surprised to find that his lungs were diseased and that the Dr. considered his case very critical." Indeed, it was so critical that the uncle died the next day.

In cookbooks, newspapers, and apothecaries, medical consumers could find a vast array of remedies to treat themselves. No matter what one's class, managing health rested on knowing when to self-medicate and when to seek professional advice. Self-medication data from diaries of middle-class patients, alongside MGH patient health histories, correspond with evidence found in daybooks of physicians discussed in chapter 1. Sources demonstrate that constipation did plague many in the Early Republic and that people in all walks of life treated themselves with cathartics or consulted private practitioners for stubborn episodes. Narcotic use by MGH patients validate data found in private practice; most patients whose medication habits were recorded show that they did not take narcotics frequently without professional consultation. When working-class patients did apply for care at the MGH, they did so for chronic diarrhea or for fevers, as hospitals could offer the bedside care and rest that might not have been available in their normal living circumstances. In the case of laborers, dressing and treatment of simple injuries, rashes, inflammation, and syphilis were more likely to be treated at home than by professionals.

Overall, MGH intake records show that patients dosed themselves with heroic remedies. Data here suggest that MGH patients were just as likely (if not more so) to treat themselves with heroic medicine as private practitioners were to prescribe them, particularly in the case of strong cathartics. This lends credence to the argument that patients' dissatisfaction with heroic care did not appear until the mid-nineteenth century. In other words, it was not that patients suffered heroic therapies meekly until new medical theories or alternative therapies could develop. Rather, they relied on heroic therapies to relieve their illnesses until the mid-nineteenth century, when their expectations of medicine changed for many reasons, including economic ones.

3
Money and Medicine

Over the course of the nineteenth century, patient sectors that could pay for medical services shifted due to a transition in economic exchange practices. This, in turn, determined who could control medical choices and, subsequently, who could shape medical therapeutics. Earlier, in the eighteenth century, medical care could be paid for through social credit, bartering, and money exchange. By 1830s, more and more physicians were demanding promissory notes or cash, especially in urban centers. Such a shift meant that certain patient populations could no longer pay and were forced into using health-care venues where they had less control over their treatments.

The economic consequences of illness also changed over time and affected patient groups differently. In the eighteenth-century home, family, servants, and field hands all could be called on to help nurse a patient or step in to perform the duties that were being neglected because of illness. If the illness persisted, the family might turn to neighbors and extended family members for advice and aid. One historian describes the social relationships created in reaction to illness in eighteenth-century New England by distinguishing between "social credit," in which "care for the afflicted was part of a system of social credits and debts" and money economy. Neighbors, family, and friends accrued social credit through favors, affection, good reputation, equipment loans, and services provided, such as nursing care. When the family decided to consult a physician, they entered into a different type of exchange. The "money" economy involved "explicit sums [that] were attached to care for the sick."[1]

As the economic relationship between physician and patient transformed over the course of the nineteenth century in urban areas, those who controlled patients' medical care altered. The commercial side of the medical relationship changed from a local exchange system to a long-distance trade system. As several economic historians have demonstrated, up until the mid-nineteenth century farmers and merchants (and physicians, I found) depended on local exchange systems. These systems measured economic performance through a long-standing trade of useful goods, services, and labor for subsistence or as payment for other debts rather than by profit. This resulted in "perpetual, complex webs of credit and debt throughout the countryside that linked households to one another."[2]

Eventually, long-distance trade systems would come to predominate in urban areas like Boston, which required regular payments in cash or promissory notes for debts. Working-class patients experienced these changes differently than did middle-to-upper-class patients. Furthermore, certain groups of working-class patients became more dependent on institutional medical care such as that offered by Massachusetts General Hospital (MGH). Ultimately, shifts in the type of economic transactions that took place between patients and their doctors influenced patient expectations and experiences of medical care.

Analysis of medical ledgers in Massachusetts demonstrate that economic exchanges between physicians and patients shifted in the Boston area beginning in the 1820s while staying relatively unchanged in rural medical practices in western Massachusetts. This reflects a broader trend seen among other commercial actors, such as farmers and merchants. The scholarship of economic historians helps to describe and explain social meanings of shifts in economic practices apparent in rural and urban physicians' daybooks and ledgers between the late eighteenth century and mid-nineteenth century in Massachusetts. Studying the social implications of physicians' use of long-distance trade systems throws light on debates over the manner and consequences of the rise of a market economy and demonstrates how changes in economic practices affected medical care.

The construction of economic activities from 1780 to 1860 can be seen as arising from changes in the interactions between the "local world of barter" and the "international network of trade" surrounding a "market economy." The three coexisted, and the boundaries between them shifted as individuals experimented and interacted with different economic practices. In other words, there was no linear progression from "altruistic and neighborly assistance to the cash nexus."[3] Yet, when cash transactions began to dominate in urban medical practices beginning in the 1820s, this had social implications for medical practice.

The fluid boundaries within the commercial relationship affected all economic sectors, including medicine. For example, shifts in economic exchanges depicted in farmers' ledgers in Massachusetts occurred in medical practices as well, transforming the medical relationship. Farmers' ledgers show that, "although the countryside took on a new dynamism, its precapitalist structure remained recognizable, even in the 1820s."[4] While advancing a "social explanation of the emergence of rural capitalism," one historian distinguishes between long-distance trade and local exchange systems, assigning each a different purpose and pattern but also discussing them in terms of different ethics.[5]

The descriptions of local exchange and long-distance trade practices provide useful tools for understanding medical relationships in the early republic. Among western Massachusetts farmers, historian Christopher Clark shows that local exchange practices persisted well into the mid-nineteenth century. For example, Amherst farmer Horace Belding's account book (1816–64) documents that he relied heavily on noncash payments. Of all his payments and receipts, 81 percent were by goods and labor and 19 percent by cash.[6] Most physicians' ledgers in the eighteenth century and *rural* physicians' ledgers in the nineteenth century reveal a similar dominance of local exchange practices in which most doctors were paid by goods, labor, and services as well as cash. As seen in farmers' and merchants' account books, medical accounts depict reciprocal financial relationships that often lasted for a lifetime.

In the eighteenth century, physicians who practiced in both urban and rural areas accepted a variety of forms of payment over long periods of time. In Westborough, Massachusetts, Colonel Nathan Fisher paid Dr. Josiah

Brigham "By making [a] Coffine for Dr. Siah" and "by honey" on January 10, 1788.[7] Dr. Edward Flint of Worcester from 1766 to 1790 was paid by weaving, spinning, beef, cider, beeswax, butter, leather, and labor of various patients' families and friends, as well as in cash.[8] Dr. John Sprague of Boston often noted the occupations of his patients as well as their payments: James Crawford, shoemaker, paid with a pair of pumps; and Temple Decoster, cabinetmaker, paid by making a desk and bookcase for Dr. Sprague.

Several patients' occupations did not coincide with their forms of payment. For instance, Mr. Agier, a silk dyer, paid with a cord of wood, and Mr. Crosby, a mason, paid with corn, demonstrating that the physician had negotiated for payments in goods that he needed or could trade. In fact, Dr. Moses Mosman of Sudbury was quite creative in exchanging his services for the wares he wanted. In May 1774, Mosman gave a gun "with an Iron Bale," "an Old Water Pole," and some medicine to Matthias Mosman and got back a gun (presumably of greater value than the one he had given) in November.[9] Before 1800, medical ledgers among urban and rural practitioners uniformly and routinely demonstrated receipt of goods, services, and labor rather than cash as payment for medical treatments and services.

Local exchange ethics meant that customers not only expected to be granted generous amounts of time to settle debts but preferred the option of paying them off by whatever means they were able. This served as a counterpoint to the ethics of long-distance trade. Although both involved reciprocity, the "local" ethic valued a reciprocity that extended over long periods of time between economic actors embedded in a social network. There was a morality in accepting obligations and discharging them over time. The local exchange ethic featured "restraint, caution, and consideration of debtors' means to pay." Pressing for settlement could cause offense by implying a lack of trust, or could be seen as an attempt to take advantage of a situation in which the balance was, at that moment, in favor of the collector.[10]

As the nineteenth century proceeded, this long-term reciprocal financial relationship began to disappear in areas around Boston. Urban practitioners came to accept noncash payments less and less often.[11] By tracing Moses Mosman's medical ledgers throughout his career, it can be demonstrated how his Sudbury practice (located twenty miles west of Boston) moved more and more toward cash or notes of hand (IOUs) as payments.[12] As table 3.1 shows, Mosman's 1763–89 accounts totaled 1,197 payment entries, of which 32 percent were by goods, services, or labor; cash accounted for

33 percent; and only 5 percent notes of hand were received. In contrast, Mosman's ledger from 1802 to 1820 confirms his shift away from accepting goods, services, and labor as payment, down 20 percent.[13]

The most dramatic change occurs in the entries "received in full" or "received in part," from 11 percent in 1763–89 to 39 percent in 1802–20. Closer scrutiny of the accounts suggests that these receipts were probably for cash at the time of the medical service; "received in full" noted payments made on or near the time of service. Payments in kind were itemized and rarely occurred at the time of service. If one accepts that "received in full or part" denotes cash payments, then the difference in the number of cash payments received from 1763–89 to 1802–20 is marked (44% to 72% respectively).

Another analytical approach reviews cash payments as a percentage of value of the total amount collected. Then an upper range would consist of interpreting "received in full" as all cash payments (fig. 1), and a lower range would consider "received in full" as including no cash. In this manner, goods and services showed a marked discrepancy in value range, 52–30 percent and 49.5–2.5 percent (1763–89 and 1802–20 respectively). The amount of increase in cash and decrease in goods and services would depend on how one interpreted "received in full." But it seems reasonable to assume that physicians became less exact (using "received in full") in recording transactions when cash became more common and transactions became less complicated by mixed payments of goods, labor, and cash.

Mosman appears to have demanded (or accepted) more notes from his patients as well (increase from 5% to 14%; table 3.1). Nathaniel Saltonstall's practice reflects a similar pattern. Practicing in Haverhill (thirty-seven miles northwest of Boston), Dr. Saltonstall received black velvet, rum, a hunting whip, and two yards of "Shalloon" from Samuel White in 1770–71, while Thomas Whittier received credit by work of Moses Clement (presumably one of Whittier's laborers) on March 22, 1782.[14] However, in the early nineteenth century, Saltonstall's ledger lists more and more notes received from patients rather than goods or labor.[15] Worcester physician Edward Flint's ledgers (1766–90 and 1795–1816) show a trend similar to Saltonstall's. Flint received steady payments in cash (50% to 49%), but a sharp decline in goods and services (32% to 16%) can be seen in table 3.2. Thus Flint shifted away from payments in goods and services to notes.

By the mid-nineteenth century, physicians' ledgers from Boston and

· CHAPTER THREE ·

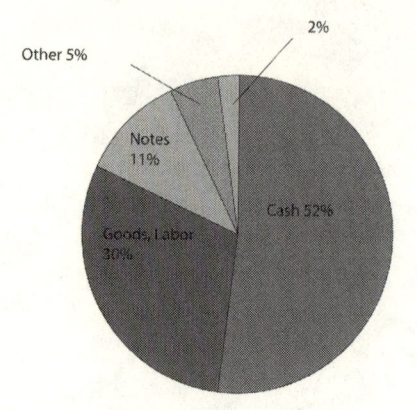

Amount Collected, 1763 to 1789 (upper range for cash)
- Cash 52%
- Goods, Labor 30%
- Notes 11%
- Other 5%
- 2%

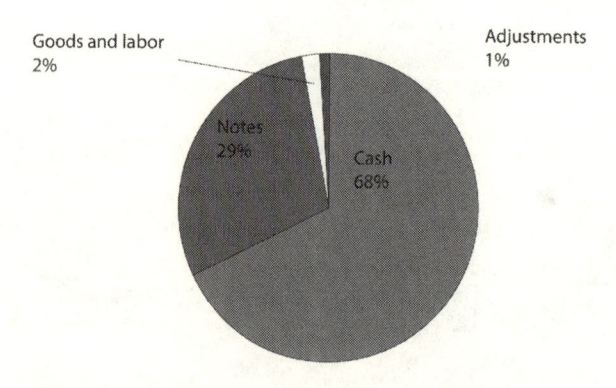

Amount Collected, 1802 to 1820 (upper range for cash)
- Cash 68%
- Notes 29%
- Goods and labor 2%
- Adjustments 1%

1763 to 1789 chart represents percentage of 420 pounds, 4 shillings, and 11 pence. 1802 to 1820 chart represents percentage of 4305.24 in dollars.

FIGURE 1. Types of payment collected by Moses Mosman, 1763–1769 and 1802–1820

Worcester became less plentiful than ledgers from surrounding rural towns. Eighteenth-century ledgers noted details of long-running accounts that doctors could consult in the event of any patients claiming to have been overcharged. Of the nineteenth-century ledgers that still exist, many lack the details (patient treatments, types of payment) that eighteenth-century ledgers uniformly contained. The demise of the long-term, local exchange system in favor of discrete cash transactions in urban areas may have meant that detailed ledgers became less necessary. Of the ledgers found, Dr. Caleb

Snow's of Boston documented almost all payments in cash, some even in advance, in his 1826 ledger.[16] Likewise, Worcester physician Benjamin F. Heywood's ledger of 1835–54 lists only payments in cash or promissory notes.[17]

One historian describes the shift to cash as a reflection of a new societal organization in which "a far greater level of economic anonymity" was achieved. The physician no longer had to base creditworthiness on his familiarity with a patient's reputation. Greater monetary liquidity "became a way to brace and control, in short, to coordinate," chains of commercial transactions among strangers in an ever larger economic space while allowing "social distance in the proximity of the neighborhood."[18] Thus the transition to cash had social ramifications. Cash did make exchanges easier, but more impersonal: the personal obligations implied in the local exchange had diminished.[19] For better and worse, the urban physician had less long-term financial ties with his patients.

After 1800, both rural and urban practitioners recorded receipt of more notes than in the eighteenth century. Although Williams's account book shows no increase in notes, other practices outside of Boston did; Flint's accounts in Worcester reveal an increase of notes by the early nineteenth century.[20] A proliferation of notes occurred especially among practices close to Boston. The number of notes jumped in Mosman's ledger from 5 percent in the 1763–89 book to 18 percent in the 1802–20 book. In terms of percentage to total value, the value of Mosman's notes increased from 11 percent to 29 percent (see figure 1).

By the early decades of the nineteenth century, the pressure for a doctor to exchange medical services for goods necessary to his household and to obtain equity given fluctuating market prices (especially on bulk produce) resulted in an increased financial insecurity in accepting goods. At the same time, payment by labor could be as slow in coming and difficult to assign a fair value as payment in goods.

Promissory notes were not completely secure either, as they represented an ambiguous exchange. The note assumed a continuing relationship between doctor and patient, as an IOU did not immediately discharge the obligation of the debtor like cash. Instead, it served as a promise to pay, one that could be sufficient enough to merit a court judgment for collection. This might have proved especially important in the case of a patient's death; the physician could collect payment from the estate with a note. In addition, the possessor of a note (the doctor) could endorse it to a third party in exchange for something of value, in which case the note functioned as cash. Accepting promissory notes rather than goods and labor allowed patients to use their credit with neighbors, which could result in a more prompt (and perhaps more secure) payment through a third party. The insistence on a note, however, signaled an alteration in the social relationship of the exchange, introducing a new tension or insecurity that prompted demand for a tangible promise of payment.[21]

The increased use of notes as payment in the nineteenth century can be seen as a transitional adaptation in the movement toward cash. In cash transactions the ethic of long-distance trade demanded quick payment: "morality lay in the quick discharge of obligation."[22] In promissory notes, the obligation remained, but for a fixed period, not as a lifelong entanglement, as was the case with the local exchange system.

In nineteenth-century rural practice, a decline of goods, services, and labor as payment and a shift to cash or notes of hand were less evident. Practitioners such as Dr. Peck in Milford, Massachusetts, recorded accepting hay, timber, and other goods and services in his 1832–34 ledger. Likewise, the practice of Dr. William Williams of Deerfield, Massachusetts, shows little change over the 1787 to 1828 period. Table 3.3 clearly reveals that Williams's patients did not shift to paying with cash or note; they continued to pay in goods, services, and labor such as tobacco, saddle or bridle work, and the castration of calves.[23] Similarly, Amos Taylor of Warwick continued to receive cords of wood, laundry services, and bushels of rye as payment well into the nineteenth century.[24]

The "precapitalist structure" of direct reciprocal exchange remained a more common form of transaction in medical practices in western Massachusetts than in practices in central Massachusetts or those surrounding Boston in the east. This geographical finding correlates with Winifred B. Rothenberg's data on farmers. Rothenberg analyzed the number and destinations of marketing trips taken by farmers in Massachusetts between 1750 and 1855 as an indicator of market concentration and, thus, market economy. In the eastern part of the state, Boston dominated as a market destination from 1791 to 1835. In the west, little market concentration in any one town occurred until 1836, when Springfield emerged as a commercial center. As with farmers, ledgers of medical practitioners demonstrate that market economy was centered in Boston in the east rather than in western Massachusetts. The ethics of local exchange in western Massachusetts persisted into the mid-nineteenth century and privileged what was best for the community over individual advancement featured in long-distance trade practices.

As Williams's practice indicates, goods, services, and labor remained the most common form of payment in rural practices. On the one hand, the persistence of payment in goods and services can be explained by the lack of coin and paper money in general. Banknotes (cash) printed by private banks became the medium of exchange, but they circulated more freely around market centers where private banks were more likely to have branches and each bank's reputation was known.[25]

Another explanation of the avoidance of cash by rural physicians can be understood as insulating "local exchanges from price fluctuations" and stimulating "production of local goods and demand for services."[26] Physicians could protect their business in locally made and sold medicines by persisting in local exchange practices. Almost all physician ledgers document the use of "proprietary" remedies, such well-known compounds as James' Fever Powder and Dover's Powder. Stephen Williams prescribed Dover's Powder frequently, as well as Johnson's Pill and Hooper's Female Pills. Patients were more likely to obtain local supplies of remedies from their local doctor, whom they could pay by goods or labor over time, than through the mail, which required immediate payment with cash.[27]

Several articles that appeared in *The Boston Medical and Surgical Journal* (*BMSJ*) provide evidence that country physicians were particularly apt to prescribe their own medicines or patent medicines. In the article "Discourse on Quackery," the author wrote that "some idea of the extent to which quack medicines are circulated may be formed by the country practitioner," who was "compelled by circumstances to carry his medicine with him, and to deal them out with his own hands." Another contributor to the *BMSJ* accused certain doctors of using patent medicines to the detriment of the profession and encouraged the practice of filling prescriptions locally. Calling himself "Gamma," he wrote that some doctors provided certificates of endorsement for quack medicines. Gamma went on to argue that physicians should cease to prescribe patent medicines because nostrum makers seldom disclosed what ingredients they contained, but as such remedies had been recommended by a physician, the public might be tempted to use them without consulting a doctor, and thus might use them improperly. Gamma advised that "if any [patent medicines] are indicated, they ought to be prepared by the exhibitor himself, or a faithful and duly qualified apothecary, to answer a particular indication in a particular case." After all, a "man of sound judgment" would make his own prescriptions rather than adhere rigidly to one formula for all cases.[28] Remedies made locally became a matter of good medical practice as well as good business. Local exchange practices would help rural physicians keep this source of income.

The social implications of shifts in payment types resulted in a greater inequity in health care among patient groups. Middle-to-upper-class patients developed less financial indebtedness to one physician, freeing them to seek simultaneous aid from various types of medical practitioners. Less-well-to-do patients, who were denied credit and had little cash, found themselves no longer able to pay promptly or in forms that were acceptable, so many were forced to find care in hospitals. Hospital care required them to forfeit certain personal freedoms, including control over medical decisions.

This is not to say that physicians did not extend free medical care to patients without cash. The form that charity took differed among physicians. One contributor to the *BMSJ* categorized collecting debts by different categories of patients. Patients who, "though honest, industrious and grateful, are, unfortunately, really unable to pay," became the most likely candidates for charity. To varying degrees, physicians' ledgers frequently record retiring debts to the "honest" poor.[29] Snow treated less fortunate patients without ever charging them. In the front cover of his 1826 medical ledger, he wrote "the charges carried out in figures are for necessary attendance and legal: those with X and blank, occasional visit & at my own discretion as such as I shall never demand."[30] One such patient, Mr. Bean, received regular visits without charge. Snow recorded visits he made to patients such as Mr. Bean only in case a medical review proved necessary. He made note of his method of leaving a blank or an X in the debit column of charitable cases to ensure that executors of his estate would not try to collect in the event of his death.

Dr. John George Metcalf's ledger shows a different approach to charitable medical care. Metcalf practiced in Mendon, Massachusetts, and its surrounding towns in Worcester County in the nineteenth century. In June 1865, he documented the reasons why specific accounts from 1845 to 1865 had remained unpaid. Presumably, he actively pursued payment and then wrote off the accounts of those patients from whom he would never receive payment. As table 3.4 shows, of the 280 accounts not paid, poverty proved to be the greatest obstacle to collecting those debts; 31 percent of the 280 patient accounts listed in the ledger did not pay in full or in part due to poverty, according to Metcalf's notations. Metcalf often designated patients as "deserving" poor, like Stephen Lesuer, whose account on May 27, 1865, was retired in the amount of $12.93 "By Honest Poverty." Metcalf voluntarily dismissed a mere 1 percent of his accounts "by [his] charity."[31] Physicians who had built less thriving practices than their urban counterparts may have needed to collect any payment offered, even from impoverished patients. However, when payment seemed unlikely, Metcalf retired the debt for those hampered by "honest" poverty.

From patients for whom debts had not been forgiven as charity, physicians more frequently demanded payment in cash or notes. Greater insecurity, partially due to movement of patients in and out of New England, prompted the increase in demands for cash and notes. For farmers, the "opportunities for advancement were comparatively limited in many areas of northeastern agriculture," which precipitated out-migration "to richer farm lands farther west or to cities in search of prospects in commerce or industry."[32] An estimated eight hundred thousand people moved from the Northeast to the West between 1790 and 1820.[33] The migration of people into cities or westward meant an influx of strangers into Boston or the possible absconding of debtors away from Massachusetts. Such large-scale movements of people in and out of the Northeast created anxiety about whether certain patients would indeed ever pay.

Discussions of problems in debt collection appeared in articles in professional magazines. In September 1845, one doctor complained that physicians were often cheated by patients who never had any intention of paying for their services. He noted that "something of this species of deception" was known in the country, "but bears no comparison to that practised [sic] in the city." In comparison, "empirics in Boston certainly conduct their affairs much more wisely than the educated faculty," because "with them it is cash down, or no prescription."[34] Another physician wrote the editor in response, suggesting that "a doctor's bill should be presented for payment—either by *cash* or *note*—quarterly [emphasis in original]." Those willing and able to pay would do so. "With the honest, industrious poor such abatement should be made, *on settlement,* as can be afforded, and an arrangement for payment of the balance suited to their condition and circumstances." As for those unwilling to pay, he suggested that doctors make a note of them in a pocket book by alphabetical index as a reminder should they ever call for medical services again.[35]

Dr. Metcalf did not collect his debts quarterly, but he did record similar problems in debt collection. Of the 30 percent of his patients who left town without settling their debts, many, among them Albert C. Bennett and Thomas S. Curtis, "went to the west." Elizabeth Rawson and other women "married out west" without paying their bills in Massachusetts. To overcome the problem of patients moving and leaving debts behind, many doctors such as Mosman, Snow, and Flint required payment through promissory notes or cash at the time of service.

Increases in payment by notes may have signaled that the medical profession wished to rectify a perceived inequity in financial security in comparison to lawyers, merchants, and mechanics. In an article titled "Profits of Medical Practice," a physician stated that fees to lawyers were regulated by law, by bar rules, or by custom "in a manner that secures to them every fraction of their dues," and merchants and mechanics in their transactions could "both require and give security, without giving offense." The intimacy of medical house calls made demands of immediate payment delicate, if not awkward. Thus, the physician "goes wherever called, not knowing whether he is to be paid or not." A doctors could be called out at any time, travel to a patient's home, and if he did not render a service, might not be paid for his time and trouble. Indeed, even if he did render a service, he still might not be paid. This way of conducting business would not be tolerated by other professions, the author claimed. Perhaps the increased use of notes was a way of to ensure that physicians would be treated as they perceived other professionals were treated.[36]

Physicians' increasing demands for cash payments altered the patient–doctor relationship. Demand for cash meant the loss of interdependence and obligation that characterized local exchange practices. In the long-distance trade relationship, urban middle-class patients, along with their disposable incomes, could partake of a widening range of healers and treatments, unhindered by the ritualized, reciprocal nature of the local exchange system. In other words, they were released from "a tangled web of debtor and creditor relationships" that lasted over a lifetime. Long-distance trade practices created formalized monetary encounters that helped establish control among strangers conducting business in an ever-widening economic space. Cash transactions meant that middle-class patients could spend their disposable income among a wider range of medical suppliers and practitioners because obligations were discharged immediately.

Certainly, patients had medical choices in the eighteenth century and in cash-poor areas in the nineteenth century. As discussed, in the eighteenth century patients consulted orthodox and irregular health givers, but they did not have alternative healers.[37] In cash-poor areas such as the rural South, alternative healers abounded: they "were everywhere and equally in hot pursuit of medical livelihood." However, as Steven Stowe argues, "a brother physician became one's toughest rival when patients narrowed their choice to the orthodox style of medicine."[38] Middle-class patients in the Boston area did not narrow their choice. Their growing disposable incomes and the ease of cash transactions allowed members of the middle class to seek care immediately and to experiment with many new treatments founded on science. The changing market offered the middle class liberating potential and expanding choices of medical services.

In the nineteenth century regular physicians bemoaned the loss of business to an ever-increasing number of alternative practitioners. Dr. J. F. Skinner wrote in *BMSJ* that there existed "so wide, varied and extensive . . . [a] range of quackery, that in considering its follies and impositions, one hardly knows where to begin or where to end. A few only of the magnitude can be here hinted at. Homoeopathic, hydropathic, electro-magnetic, botanic, mesmeric, and Indian, all come in for a share." Dr. J. L. Chandler speculated that the amount of money paid for various nostrums "undoubtedly exceeds the sum paid to physicians for their services. In our cities, probably, the balance in favor of the *trade* is still greater." Add to this the fee "exacted by mountebanks of every sort, from the impudent mesmerizer down to the hypocritical or fanatical homoeopathist, and the proportion of compensation to the regular physician dwindles to an insignificant pittance." Later, Chandler imagined that half their pittance actually came from those whose health had been ruined by mountebanks. He claimed that one of his patients had paid him six dollars for treatment one year while spending five to six hundred on other treatments.

Whether or not Chandler was indulging in hyperbole, he and other physicians wrote regularly to their professional journals about business they lost to various treatments that "burst upon the world, like a flaming meteor." Many physicians witnessed medical fads that came "with their signs out," their "flaming handbills" posted everywhere advertising lectures and demonstrations, only to disappear again, leaving "[their] advocates and those . . . [they] had deceived in utter darkness and dismay."[39] The medical market provided a plethora of choices for the unfettered disposable income of the middle class.

Wealthy patients also utilized notes in order to preserve their cash reserves; payment in promissory notes eased problems with uneven cash supplies. But of course promissory notes relied on the creditworthiness of an individual. Acceptance of a note as payment for medical services would require the physician's familiarity with a patient's reputation. Itinerant laborers, who could no longer pay in goods or labor, lacked the reputation in the community required to pay by promissory note. A switch to payments in cash or notes meant that these workers who moved in and out of the community could receive medical care only in hospitals or almshouses.

One historian described the almshouse as "the hospital of last resort." And no wonder, for it housed paupers from a variety of backgrounds and conditions of health. A warehouse of disparate and desperate people, the almshouse contained the intemperate, the insane, the chronically ill, the incurable, and the contagious—none of whom received much medical care.[40]

Created to be an antithesis of the almshouse, Massachusetts General Hospital (MGH) opened its doors in 1821 to serve deserving Americans whose poverty existed through no fault of their own, usually as a result of illness. The MGH ostensibly did not treat contagious or chronically ill patients, but hospital records show that this rule was difficult to enforce. Patients who sought treatment at MGH were asked to supply a written application that was then reviewed by the attending physician, who either accepted or denied admission. The visiting committee (a rotating delegation of the Board of Trustees) would determine whether the patient was considered fit to remain and if any fee would be charged. Emergency cases could circumvent this process but would be approved retroactively.[41]

Whether they received treatment in the almshouse or hospital, therapeutic decisions made in physician-dominated hospital wards or almshouses decreased patients' ability to negotiate decisions about their treatments.[42] Paupers could not be choosers. Significantly, cash-poor patients who resided in the community and in earlier days had been able to pay for medical treatments in goods and services over time could no longer do so. Those with a decent reputation, however, might sign a promissory note or obtain home treatment through the Boston Dispensary if recommended by a subscriber.

Treatment through the Boston Dispensary meant that the patient received care at home, or at least in familiar surroundings.[43] The dispensary provided each patron with two tickets of admission for every five dollars they contributed. They could then select sick persons they felt worthy of their charity to receive free medical remedies and visits at home.[44] Thus, cash-poor patients who enjoyed some social credit could receive care at home through the Boston Dispensary.

As choices in acceptable payment options shrank, more and more laborers were forced into the MGH wards. The records of MGH demonstrate the social implications of the move to cash transactions and long-distance trade practice for working-class patients. As the "Occupational Classification Table" (table 3.5) demonstrates, the category that showed the most marked rise in admittance to MGH occurred among the "Semiskilled and Services" (21%, 42%, and 39%, in the 1820s, 1830s, and 1840s, respectively). It is among the semiskilled and services occupations that the transition to cash had the greatest effect.

Domestics accounted for a large portion of the semiskilled and services group, those seeking care from the hospital rising from 7 percent in the 1820s to 22 percent in the 1840s. Prescriptive literature often including topics on how to manage illness among servants shows the centrality of illnesses of domestics as a key societal concern. In *Domestic Duties* (1828), Frances Parkes encouraged young wives not to send their sick servants home to "poor, confined, and dirty lodgings," but to care for them in the comfort of their master's house, attended by healthy servants, who "should be encouraged to pay as much attention as their time will permit." Although Parkes considered it cruel to send servants to the hospital, she tempered her opinion by saying that it was not her intent to "object to hospitals in general; on the contrary, there are many cases that could not receive the same degree of attention, or have such advantages in medical consultation, as in the hospital." Parkes criticized only those employers who sent their domestics from "habitations of splendor and luxury, into such dissimilar scenes" when their constitutions were at their lowest level of health. Parkes believed that medical care should be paid for by employers, not by deduction from wages.[45] Yet, data from MGH suggest that employers increasingly did not heed the advice of Parkes on this matter. The semiskilled and domestics population could not barter for medical services, did not have abundant cash reserves, or possess the social credit to attain recommendation for the dispensary's at-home care. As a result more and more patients from this occupational category sought care from MGH.

Patients under the categories of "Professional," "Commercial-Proprietor," and "Commercial-Employees" showed little or decreasing change in their use of the hospital. Professionals may well have become impoverished due to their illnesses, such as a fifty-four-year-old former physician who in 1823 sought care at the MGH for constipation; he reported that he had given up his profession five years previously due to paralysis.[46] But most of these people were more likely to have connections to wealthy people who were able to extend charity to them or, at the very least, were subscribers to the dispensary. Former attorneys, clergy, merchants, grocers, bookkeepers, and clerks who suffered prolong illnesses eventually would have limited medical choices, but they would still retain some agency through their social credit. In other words, one imagines that if they were displeased with their care, they still might possess enough influence to damage a physician's reputation with well-placed complaints. In contrast, semiskilled patients who could no longer barter for medical services and who were admitted to MGH had very little control over their medical care other than to leave. In 1849 a seventeen-year-old male admitted for pain in his side chose to "elope" (a term used to indicate a person who left without consent or against advice) the next day. Although the house physician did not record why the young man had left, he did record that he was "intolerably stupid."[47] Few patients chose to leave.

Occupational designation represents only one factor influencing medical care. The marital status and gender of a patient also determined what medical care, if any, a person received. House physicians recorded more single patients (both male and female) than married ones. Surprisingly, widowed women did not constitute a large proportion of the population in the hospital ward in any of the decades studied. Impoverished widows may have been "worthy" candidates for benevolence from private-practice physicians or for aid from the dispensary.[48] A widow's worthiness could be offset by her behavior, however, as one fifty-four-year-old widow in 1825 demonstrates. The MGH house physician recorded that her husband had died last June, which affected her very much ("rendered her melancholy"). This in turn aggravated a preexisting disorder of rheumatism and inflammation of the eyes, and she had grown increasingly feeble. But the dispensary was not likely to provide her with aid given that she had "a strong desire for drink," "indulged herself in drinking wine—spirit—coffee—tea—&c in considerable quantities." In fact, the woman admitted to the doctor that she was "very foolish & has come here that she may get rid of her bad habits, & be made to do as she out [*sic*] to."[49]

Patients in their twenties and thirties found medical care through benevolence and charity particularly hard to obtain. Hospitals such as the MGH emerged to fill such gaps in health care. In 1810, Drs. James Jackson and James C. Warren prepared a circular letter addressed to wealthy Bostonians outlining the need for the hospital. While the dispensary treated hundreds of patients who could afford food and housing but not medical bills, the almshouse was inadequate both as a house of correction and as a hospital. The MGH strove to provide care so that industrious young workers who are "deserving objects of charity" would not have to languish in the almshouse among "the worst members of the community, the debauched and the profligate."[50] Patient records at the MGH confirm that those admitted for treatment were young: the mean age of MGH patients fell between twenty-eight to thirty years old from the 1820s to the 1840s.[51] The MGH was established to treat those who were industrious but had not yet had a chance to accumulate enough wealth to weather a bout of illness.

Frequently, foreign-born patients became patients in the hospital. Seventy-one percent of patients whose country of origin was documented and who were admitted between 1823 and 1849 hailed from Ireland, the majority of whom had been in the country less than five years. Occupations that normally would earn greater social credit, such as the legal profession, could be offset by factors such as country of origin and number of years in residency. For example, a thirty-year-old lawyer from Ireland had come to the United States fourteen months prior to falling ill. With no solid ties to the community, his receiving benevolence from either a private-practice physician or the Boston Dispensary would seem unlikely. The MGH provided care for such worthy but unconnected patients.[52]

Wealth alone was not the sole criterion for whether patients retained their medical agency. Other factors such as age, occupation, gender, ethnicity, and number of years' residence in Boston influenced each patient's social credit or ability to negotiate care. When economic practices changed from barter to cash transactions, it was not those in the poorest ranks who were the most affected, but the working, semiskilled young person. In an increasingly industrialized urban center, this group of infirmed patients began to overload hospitals.

In sum, the decrease in long-term reciprocal financial obligations between physicians and patients in urban practices resulted in a decrease in financial indebtedness, altering the nature of the patient–physician relationship. In contrast, rural physicians continued receiving payments in goods, labor, and services. An adherence to bartering practices meant that nineteenth-century rural physicians could insulate themselves from sharp price fluctuations while protecting their pharmaceutical businesses; patients who lacked cash could obtain their medicines from local doctors who accepted labor, services, or goods as payment rather than purchasing ready-made medicines from proprietary drug sellers who required cash payments.

In urban medical practice, the shift to mainly cash transactions had social implications. Patients belonging to "professional," "commercial-proprietor," and "commercial-employee" occupation categories, as well as "skilled" tradesmen who lacked cash, could no longer pay with goods and labor. Those who lived in the community and had established creditworthiness could make medical payments with promissory notes. If they possessed enough social credit, they could be provided medical care through the benevolence of subscribers to the Boston Dispensary. Otherwise, they too had to depend on institutional health care or the mercy of a physician for medical treatment. The truly poor had always had to rely on charitable organizations such as almshouses. Those affected most by changing economic exchange practices were those who performed semiskilled and service-oriented jobs. For specific urban working sectors, medical negotiations became more limited with the loss of bartering practices.

However, the movement to cash payments was not detrimental to everyone. For urban doctors, cash payment allowed more financial security in a credit culture that included more and more strangers. For middle-class patients, the change to discrete cash transactions offered an opportunity to seek a cure among a variety of practitioners. Thus, changes in economic practices limited medical choices for some patient groups and expanded choices for others. Over the course of the early nineteenth century, cash-paying (or at least note-worthy) patients exerted more influence on medical care through their choices than did their cash-poor counterparts. Whether such patients expected to *find* a cure among medical treatments depended on their religious beliefs.

4
Patient Expectations and Religious Beliefs

Twelve-year-old Louisa Trumbull of Worcester, Massachusetts, wrote faithfully in her diary about her brother Johnny's struggle with "dropsy [edema] on the chest." On February 7, 1833, her family had "committed to the earth" their "little darling Johnny." In recording the illness of her younger brother, Louisa inadvertently highlighted a key issue concerning religion and illness. As Johnny's condition worsened, his mother had told him that Dr. Green would give him medicine to make him better. In a momentary recuperation, "when he got so he could lisp his prayer," his mother explained to him that "God had made him better and that he must be very thankful." Apparently, the boy had given her statement some thought and one night raised himself up in his bed and said, "Mother, I say Dr. Greene is not God!"[1]

In the end, of course, neither Dr. Greene nor God cured Johnny. But Johnny's confusion about the role God played in illness mirrored that of contemporary adults. Did God cause disease as a punishment for sin, or did illness result from secular causes? Did God cure, or did doctors? The ways in which individuals answered these questions can be understood in the context of a shifting nineteenth-century religious landscape that changed patient expectations of medical care.

Changing perceptions of illness during the early nineteenth century were not necessarily a process of secularization, as some historians have argued, but more a shift in religious beliefs.[2] The increasing interest in science did not mark a decline in piety; the relationship between science and religion was not a dichotomous one. Rather, within various religious denominations the emphasis on each of the "three great symbolic centers" of Christianity—God, humanity, and nature—altered. Evidence found in diaries, correspondence, and journals shows that patients closely identified with religious values and held deep-rooted concerns for their spiritual selves, but whether they believed pain and illness were acts of God, and to what degree a man's (or a doctor's) actions could cure them, depended on their specific religious beliefs. Examples among orthodox Congregationalists, Unitarians, revivalists, and transcendentalists demonstrate that there was a spectrum of attitudes regarding God's role in illness. The belief in special providences across various denominations appears to be a general indicator of what expectations patients held for their treatment and recovery in the Early Republic.

Until roughly 1800, diaries and letters written by residents of New England who were struggling with ailments, both acute and chronic, had often expressed a desire to be relieved of pain. These authors voiced expectations of all-out cure less frequently than their mid-nineteenth-century counterparts.[3] When used by orthodox physicians or patients in the eighteenth century, "cure" designated a treatment rather than a promise to eradicate an illness.[4] As the nineteenth century unfolded, an expectation of "cure" meaning the complete eradication of disease emerged; the significance of illness and pain altered; and medical experimentation among patients across various religious denominations abounded.

As an illustration of the evolution of the language of cure, Justus Forward, an ordained minister in Belchertown, Massachusetts, for fifty-six years provides a typical example of an eighteenth-century person's approach to therapeutics. Forward struggled to help his father, Joseph, who was suffering from an unspecified, prolonged illness, and described that help in terms of relief rather than cure.[5] On February 10, 1766, Forward wrote in his journal, "My father had sent for me and was at the point of Death . . .

he had the bilious colic & gravel had been extreme ill but the Extremity of pain was removed before I got there." In a March 24 entry, it becomes clear that his father was being treated by physician. "Father was more easy—this perhaps owing to opiates."[6] Throughout his father's illness, Forward documented favorable results in terms of his father being "more easy," "comfortable," and having his pain "removed." By April, Forward wrote that his father "appeared resigned to Gods will & not anxious about Life or Death, he gave us good Reason to think he was interested in Christ & had a good Hope himself."[7]

Forward's language of relief is echoed in other New England journals, such as that of Rebecca Dickenson of Hatfield, Massachusetts, who documented her desire to be eased or relieved in her diary entry of November 15, 1787: "[A cold] has confined me for a week with the most distressing Collick thought my life to be going—the day of my illness sent for Dr. Williams who opened a vein which has given me ease."[8] On June 8, 1783, Anna Sophia Brigham sent a letter to Josiah Brigham regarding his sister's health: "She is much as she was when you saw her. I think her cough seem[s] to be Mitigated a Little. I can't say she is really any better. . . . I hope Doct. Stimson will be Able to Administer something for her relief."[9]

Physicians likewise discussed treatments in the language of relief. John Syng Dorsey described Isabel Mathews's treatment on February 9, 1805. She was suffering from a swollen abdomen, pain in her side, and a swollen, painful right leg. He treated her with a bolus to purge her and a blister to reduce her pain. On February 13, he noted, "pains not at all relieved." After prescribing a draught, he recorded that she "was relieved by the draught last night got some sleep & feels ye whole easier today."[10]

Dr. Hugh Lenox Hodge of Philadelphia succinctly expressed relief as a central expectation of patients and a goal of physicians when he recorded: "The chief of the moral qualities peculiarly required of a Physician is Humanity; That Sensibility of Heart that makes us feel for the Distress of our Fellow Creatures, and which of consequence incites us in the most powerful manner to relieve them. . . . The Patient feels his Approach like that of a Guardian Angel ministering to his Relief —Gregory."[11] A doctor who possessed "Humanity" recognized physical distress in his patients and considered it his duty to provide them with relief.

As one scholar noted, New Englanders often expressed illness in terms of "finding" one in sickness or health as a way of "mapping the location of bodies that moved continually through space and into and out of health. Finding conveyed a sense of discovery, an inquiry into a matter over which one had little control."[12] Thus, eighteenth-century patients (and their physicians) expressed expectation in terms of relief while they waited to see if the body moved into a state of health. If they used the term "cure," they meant treatment, not a demanded outcome.[13] The use of heroic treatments such as cathartics (even mild-to-moderate-acting types) in the late eighteenth century into the early nineteenth century gave visible signs of change in the ill. "The physician, patient, and patient's family could all witness and appreciate the simple fact that it was working," and the appearance of some change must have proved comforting.[14]

Religious views of illness could offer some sense of control and comfort amid struggles for good health. Hannah Heaton of North Haven, Connecticut, exemplified the eighteenth-century religious attitude toward affliction. On December 18, 1785, she fretted that her husband would never be healed: "My husband told me that there was a hard lump agrowing [sic] on his cheek. He went to a doctor but means seems [sic] to do no good. The lump grows bigger fast it is now as big as a dollar and very hard. But o but o how secure and stupid his mind is he goes on in his old ways of sinning not the least reformation. . . . Lord i believe if thou wilt thou canst make him clean and o that thou would heal his body."[15] Her despair was not directed at the physician or his treatment but at her husband, who would not change his sinful ways. In the face of her husband's lack of piety, Heaton exerted the only control she felt she had—she prayed.

Others found meaning in their illnesses. Experience Richardson of Sudbury, Massachusetts, in 1765 pondered: "God often brings me into affliction and then delivers me out again & this is a wise way of trying me for it makes me humble & thankfull."[16] Richardson saw her afflictions as instructive—as making her more appreciative of God's graces. Similarly, Rebecca Dickinson, as a strict Calvinist, viewed her sickness as evidence of God's attention and as an opportunity to show her fealty to Him: "i have Plead with god for health but Sickness is my Portien[.] gods will must Stand and i would Sing of mercy for it is good to be sick[.] it is good to be afflicted for thereby i have learned to keep thy Commands."[17]

Diaries like Heaton's, Richardson's, and Dickinson's exemplify the ways in which patients' religious beliefs helped them to place illness in their lives. Their religious convictions also influenced their expectations of medical care. In the eighteenth century, New Englanders could "entertain both providential and mechanistic explanations of illness; not every malady was understood to be related to sin (at least not as its proximate cause)."[18] In other words, a cold soaking in the rain could be seen as having caused a loved one's illness rather than his sinful nature. Nevertheless, for many patients, cure was God's gift, and promises of cure came only from itinerant healers who peddled their nostrums from town to town.[19]

In the closing decades of the eighteenth century, Enlightenment ideals increasingly challenged the traditional Protestant understanding of the relationship between pain and piety and subsequently altered patients' expectations of medical remedies and services among certain Christians. Pain came to be seen as more secular, according to historian Elaine Crane, to the "extent that the medical profession had begun to concentrate on nerve and muscle function and scientific experimentation."[20] Physicians became interested in pain as a sign of disease.

By 1809, when physician Jacob Porter began practicing medicine in Plainfield, Massachusetts, he discussed patients sometimes in terms of cure and at others in terms of relief. "Abner Fobes of Buckland, between 17 and 18 years of age, applied to me on account of a cutaneous eruption on his forehead," Porter recorded on October 30, 1809, and went on to quote Fobes's description of the outbreak: "In warm weather it rages, to use his own expression, so as to be very troublesome." Fobes described the progression of his condition from the previous spring, when "he was troubled with dizziness and extreme headache" and "the pimples on his forehead are not large but thick." Porter prescribed Fowler's solution of arsenic and on November 18 declared that Fobes's forehead contained "scracily [sic] the appearance of a pimple and the cure may be considered complete."[21]

Like many patients, Fobes consulted Porter due to the worsening of pain over a long duration.[22] Lowell Robinson suffered a painful headache for a year, but only when it "was quite troublesome, so as sometimes to keep him from labor" did he confer with a physician.[23] In these cases, neither Fobes nor Robinson perceived any cause for their ailment, and both seemed satisfied with periods of relief. The application of sulfuric ether to the forehead and other treatments achieved relief on several occasions, with a few relapses of headache noted as well.[24] In May 1810, Olive Packard suffered a dull pain in her stomach for two or three years before finding relief in Dr. Porter's remedies. In fact, for twelve months beginning in December

1809, Porter almost daily recorded his patients' conditions, in his words and theirs, as well as the outcome of his treatments. Of the thirty-three patients he treated over the course of a year, Porter used terms such as "good relief," "no relief," and "much relieved" twenty-three times, while using the term "cured" only seven.

Unfortunately, Porter's extensive notes on one year of practice were not replicated by his contemporaries. However, his records do reflect a pattern seen in many journals of both patients and doctors in which the word "relief" was common compared to the use of the word "cure." Of course, Porter's recording of his patients' use of the word "relief" may have been influenced by the questions he asked; he does not document whether he questioned them or not. Regardless, Porter's records serve as useful examples. No physician or patient suddenly ceased to use the word "relief" and replaced it with the word "cure" as an outcome of medical treatment; rather, the meaning and frequency of use of the word "cure" changed gradually over time.

Dr. James Jackson, Sr., of Boston lamented the change in the meaning of "cure" when he wrote to his son in 1833:

> [I] never fall into the error of believing that I cure (in the common sense of the word) any larger proportion of my patients. I do not like this use of the word cure—this prejudiced sense of it. For it is a very good word in its proper sense & I do not know any substitute—accordingly in my lects [sic] I always state that it is derived from *cura*—the physician shd [sic] take care of the sick—he is or should be more capable of this than other persons—but he s[hould] not undertake by drugs to overcome all their dis[ease]s.[25]

In Jackson's opinion, "cure" had changed from the "proper sense" of its meaning—to treat a disease or patient—to a "prejudiced sense" of it in which patients expected the physician to "overcome" disease.

Louisa Park's journal reflects the expectations for the elimination of disease that Jackson dismissed. When Dr. John Park left to serve as assistant surgeon aboard the USS *Warren*, he encouraged his wife to keep a journal for amusement and to provide "an interesting manuscript for my perusal should it please Providence to permit my safe return."[26] Louisa Park faithfully documented events, including the illness of their son, Warren. On Monday, April 13, 1800, the child experienced a great deal of pain from swellings under his chin and ear. Fearing that her son was suffering from scrofula, Park went to Newburyport to seek advice from friends as to which physician to consult. "They advised me to apply to Dr. Broadstreet, as having made some cures of the kind," she wrote. On examination, Broadstreet said that the swelling was a tumor, but "not of the worst kind" and that "he believed he could cure him."[27]

Park recorded that the medicines Broadstreet prescribed "appeared to operate too severely, or else the child was much worse." By Wednesday April 15, the other side of the child's neck and ear had begun to swell rapidly, and on Saturday a violent fever overtook him, he had "an inclination to puke," and his breathing became so difficult he was "groaning in agony for breath." Park documented her distress, "I was frightened—called a boy and sent him to Newburyport for Dr. Broadstreet, With all the haste possible." At nine o'clock he came and gave an emetic. It relieved the boy some and "prevented immediate suffocation."[28]

As her son appeared to be better, Park did not send for the doctor the next day. By nightfall, she came to regret that decision: the child had grown worse. On Monday morning he suffered so much that she hastily sent for the doctor. There was "the appearance of death" on his face and he seemed to be "in the agonies of death." In a desperate attempt, the doctors prescribed poultices for the child's feet, a blister for his whole breast, a strong mercurial ointment on his throat, and they gave him "calomel—antimony when necessary—lemonade with salt of tartar." But to no avail. They "pronounced him a dead child." Louisa wrote:

> I forced myself out of the chamber, & throwing myself on the bed, gave vent to the agonies of my soul. I wept and prayed until I became more composed, and then returned to the chamber, to hear the last sobs and close the eyes of my only son. For hours, I had wished to see him quiet; but when the time came I thought my own breath would have stopped. No one, that never felt can conceive the distress of such a situation. For me to describe is impossible—I will not attempt it.[29]

Louisa prayed for composure, not for cure. She sought, was promised, and expected a cure from her physicians. Instead, she experienced the death of her only son, Joseph Warren Park.

In the nineteenth century, the expectation that therapeutic outcomes should, and could, provide a cure for common illnesses became more prevalent among the growing middle class due to an increasing confidence in science and a shift in religious beliefs.[30] By the mid-nineteenth century, the development of organ and cellular pathology in Germany and clinical work in Edinburgh that demonstrated a connection between lesions in specific areas of the brain and physical disorders contributed to the growing confidence in science. Through experimentation and observation, scientists began to view the ailing body as a machine that could be fixed. These developments fostered a new optimism that, through science, man could have more control over illness.[31]

In concert with promising physiological discoveries, evolved religious views repositioned God's role in pain and sickness. In the eighteenth century, "American ministers preached that pain stemmed from original sin and that it was God's method of behavior modification. God meted out pain for two reasons: to test the faithful and offer them the opportunity to exhibit spiritual excellence or as a direct reproach for sin."[32] During the early nineteenth century, theological shifts contributed to patients' expectations in which patients sought an eradication of disease through men's actions rather than God's will.

Theologians ruminated on the contradictions between man's free will and God's role in the world, known as the concept of Providence.[33] The range of beliefs concerning free will or providential control spanned from deists, who believed solely in free will, to conservatives, who insisted that God had exclusive control. Most theologians struggled to find answers in the middle ground. New England ministers divided God's actions in the world into general providences, miracles, and special providences. General providences referred to God's natural laws; these operated without any special divine intervention. Miracles designated God's direct interference with the natural laws in order to demonstrate His divine power. Special providences proved to be the most difficult to discern because of their obscure nature. They were God's subtle messages to man in the form of events that might appear to have been brought about by natural laws but were, in fact, special acts of God.[34] Special providences included the role of illness and pain as God's message to an individual. Christians viewed sickness as an opportunity to improve one's spiritual health or as a painful reminder that God kept track of one's sins. Whether they believed illness was an example of God's special providence or not influenced patients and their expectations of medical care.

In the Massachusetts religious landscape, Congregationalism held significant ground. Congregationalists in nineteenth-century Massachusetts such as Deborah Vinal Fiske show us the traditional attitude of Congregationalism toward illness. Sheila Rothman argues that "in Deborah's value system, religious conviction took precedence over medical prescription."[35] Fiske worshipped at the Park Street Church, one of Boston's most orthodox Congregational churches in 1825. She married Nathan Fiske, a graduate of the Andover Theological Seminary, which opened its doors in protest at the appointment of a Unitarian as president of Harvard. Like a more traditional Congregationalist, Fiske would have rejected liberal Protestants' emphasis on rationalism.

Traditional Congregationalists continued to understand salvation as a gift from God to the elect, those He had already chosen to save. Congregationalists did not believe there were any actions that could be taken to earn grace. Yet, a congregant should be prepared to undergo a conversion experience, a divine revelation that an individual was part of the elect. As Congregationalists waited for God's sign of their salvation, in illness they waited for His cure.

Within this religious framework, Deborah Fiske struggled with consumption that often left her an invalid.[36] She educated herself about her condition by reading medical texts and corresponded with other sufferers from consumption, sharing remedies for pain. She wrote to Ann Schofield, "Your disease is one which I don't pretend to understand so you will escape any old woman 'certain cures,' but I have had it myself.... All these medical technicals are like so much Greek to me, and I am willing they should remain so unless I could make such knowledge a means of relief to somebody."[37] Her placement of quotation marks around "certain cures" suggests that she questioned the idea of cure promised by irregular healers while sincerely wishing she had a means of relief to offer her friend.

Fiske wrote a letter to her husband, Nathan, that reveals her position on God's role in disease:

> Friday I had quite a sick day.... I had a severe headache & considerable pain. In the evening Dr. Warren came & said it was only owing to the accumulation of phlegm & that an emetic would relieve me. I took one immediately, it operated well & I have since been better.... Independence & pride & vanity & self complacency have been at the root of every thing I have done & I have found more happiness in being constantly busy with any lawful employment than in growing in the knowledge of God & relying on the Savior for salvation; but now I am as it were laid aside & I know you will pray that the time

which is thrown upon my hands may be spent in preparing for a better home.[38]

Fiske thought she had derived too much happiness from her busy activities rather than pursuing her knowledge of God, and now God had given her an opportunity, through her incapacitating illness, to prepare her soul for heaven. Two days later, she reiterated her view of God's role in her world when she stated that they should go about "cheerfully to do our duty & leave all results with God."[39]

Fiske managed her condition as a "wary and sophisticated consumer of medicine," but did so abiding by conservative religious and domestic beliefs and using orthodox medicine. Dr. Gridley treated her while she resided in Amherst, and she often consulted or corresponded with Dr. John Collins Warren, and, in the last stages of her illness, with Dr. James Jackson—all regular physicians.[40]

For the most part, Congregational churches of eastern Massachusetts, including those in Boston, had shifted from the orthodoxy of Puritan Calvinists to Unitarianism by the early nineteenth century. Unitarians may never have succeeded in accruing any large numbers outside of New England but "they enjoyed an intellectual influence far out of proportion to their actual numbers."[41] In other words, their influence as writers meant that Unitarian leaders held sway beyond the borders of Massachusetts.

Unitarians retained the emphasis on moral living and the duty and sense of responsibility to society but dismissed the need for spiritual transformation by God's supernatural grace in order to be saved. In other words, they believed that one saved oneself by living rightly, not through a conversion experience. Unlike old Calvinists, Unitarians did not stress the sinful depravity of humans but believed in a universal moral code by which everyone should live.

Unitarians have been described as the intellectual heirs of liberal Protestantism, advanced by theologians such as Charles Chauncy, pastor of First Church; Jonathan Mayhew, pastor of West Church—both of Boston; and Ebenezer Gay, pastor of the Congregationalist church, First Parish, in Hingham, Massachusetts. Chauncy pronounced that religious conversion was an internal process characterized by how one lived one's life, not by potentially deceptive public (and emotional) conversions such as those of the First Great Awakening of the 1740s and 1750s. Gay called for a "supernatural rationalism" in response to the revival of Calvinist doctrines espoused by the evangelical preachers. With supernatural rationalism, Gay attempted to place concepts of the Enlightenment within a religious framework that included a Christian revelation where some truths existed above reason. Liberal Protestants believed that truth could be found in human reason as well as in God's revelation.[42]

Building on the theology of Chauncy, Gay, and others, Unitarians laid claim to the Congregational churches throughout Boston and its surrounding areas by the early nineteenth century, especially after the appointment in 1808 of Unitarian Samuel Webber as president of Harvard, one of the foremost schools of theology in United States. As historian Daniel Walker Howe described it, Harvard Unitarianism represented "the classic Unitarian world view" in which an integrated theology, "a confluence of Protestantism with the Enlightenment," was created.[43] Among the greatest Unitarian voices were those of Joseph Stevens Buckminster, pastor of the Brattle Street Church in Boston, and his successor in 1812, Dr. William Ellery Channing.[44]

Famously, in 1819 Channing delivered the "Unitarian Christianity" sermon, declaring the beliefs of Unitarians. Most Unitarians rejected the historic Christian belief in the divinity of Christ. In other words, they did not believe in the Holy Trinity—only God was divine. They did not view humans as inherently sinful either. Channing argued that to believe that God brought humans into the world wholly depraved, with the propensity for evil acts, would be cruel and tantamount to the "most merciless despotism." Similarly, Unitarians rejected the idea of an elect, the belief that "God selected from this corrupt mass a number to be saved." It seemed unreasonable to expect "the rest of mankind, though left without that special grace," nevertheless to repent. Important to Unitarians' perception of medicine was how they understood God's role in the world: "If God be infinitely wise, he cannot sport with the understandings of his creatures." In Channing's view, God was not in the habit of toying with his creations. Like a wise teacher, God could be found "adapting himself to the capacities of his pupils," not attempting to perplex them with "what is unintelligible," not "distressing them with apparent contradictions, not in filling them with skeptical distrust of their own powers."[45] Channing and the Unitarians did not believe that God made his lessons obscure.

Nineteenth-century Unitarians believed in general providence (natural laws) and miracles (the obvious break from natural laws) but did not place much emphasis on special providences (God's lessons hidden in ordinary events). Illness signaled a disruption of natural laws, and each patient could avoid disease by "living rightly"—both spiritually and physically. Unitarian preachers separated nature from God and "exalted the human capacity for self-determination."[46] Unitarians had faith that they could and should seek cures as well as take preventative measures because humans have free will and control; they were not fatalistic.[47]

Written in the mid-nineteenth century, Daniel F. Child's diaries exemplify the rational influences on Unitarians' views about illness. The Childs became active members of their Unitarian church. His wife taught Sunday school, and they attended the celebrations of the Suffolk Street Chapel Sunday School.[48] They kept abreast of the proceedings of the Boston Association of Unitarian Ministers as well as the Unitarian Convention in Salem in 1847.[49] As Unitarians, the members of the Child family would have sought help for pain in many different ways, not viewing it as a test of spirit or a rebuke for sin. Pain or illness was met with active resistance, not passive endurance.

Daniel Child prided himself on attending lectures and educating himself about the latest medical techniques. On January 6, 1843, Daniel, his wife, and his sister-in-law went to "a party of some twenty five persons to witness the effect of animal magnetism. Mr. Daniel Ford, our neighbor, magnetized his wife, Mary, who it is said, easily yields to the influence of this mysterious power." On another occasion, Mr. Child attended a lecture given by an "electric" physician: "Evening, husband attended the fifth lecture of Doct. Paige. Subjects—Electricity, Galvanism, and Magnetism—each briefly explained and demonstrated. Electricity declared to be the sole power of matter. The tooth ache and headache cured before the audience."[50]

Child became so confident about his knowledge of galvanism after hearing several lectures that on April 23, 1849, he recorded: "Evening charged the galvanic battery, recently bought of Dr. Paige, and applied it to all the members of the family, through the arms &c. The children were very shy in taking hold of the wires."[51] The Childs actively pursued knowledge of the latest scientific experimentation, including electric therapy. Although Robert Hare, MD, professor of chemistry at the Medical Department of the University of Pennsylvania, explored the presence of an electric fluid in the body that worked primarily on the nervous system as a field of study, the use of electricity as a curative could provoke charges of quackery, or at least was considered highly questionable by orthodox physicians. Yet Child embraced new medical treatments and eagerly experimented with various practitioners to maintain good health, apparently much to the chagrin of his children.[52]

Daniel Child's experimentation with the newest medical trends did not mean that he shunned more orthodox treatments. He frequently consulted several practitioners simultaneously. Often suffering with pain in the groin or the small of his back, he received care from Zabdiel Adams with emetics and opium, from Paige with "an application of galvanism," and from William Wesselhoeft with "a homeopathic treatment" to prevent pain.[53] For example, on August 23, 1849, Child suffered from another attack of pain in the small of his back. In the morning, he "called on Doct. Paige and had an application of electro magnetism," and in the evening he went back to taking nitric acid, which Dr. Adams had prescribed.[54] Thus Child used several physicians and several remedies as part of his responsibility to keep himself healthy. Although he wrote of religious matters, he never evoked God's name as a cause of or a cure for illness, suggesting that he did not relate his physical ailments to God's actions.

The diaries of Lucy Chase of Worcester offer another example of the influence of Unitarianism on a patient's medical choices and expectations. Although she was raised a Quaker, Chase became strongly influenced by Unitarianism.[55] Like Child, she sought cures from many types of medical practitioners. In 1842, she became curious about magnetism: "Went to Uncle M's this evening. Dr. Collyer was there, he magnetized Martha & performed a variety of experiments upon her, had her examine his chest, prescribe for Elisabeth & Sarah Folger & taste a variety of articles."[56] She attended several of Dr. Cutler's lectures on anatomy and physiology at the Mechanic Association.[57] Chase also consulted a leading orthodox physician in town, a Dr. Green, and sought the advice of noted phrenologist Orson Squire Fowler.

Lucy Chase displayed the same political activism, medical experimentation, and curiosity as the Child family. Both Child and Chase, as members of the middle class and as Unitarians, believed that human actions could effect change. "From the Lowell Institute in Boston, where crowds of 2,000 gathered to hear Benjamin Silliman's chemistry lectures, to the countless lyceums directed by local clergyman and doctors," citizens like them actively pursued scientific knowledge and felt confident that when one was ill, knowledge and experimentation could find answers that would lead toward a cure.[58]

However, all Unitarians did not share the same points of view, especially in the early decades of the nineteenth century. After all, Unitarian preachers did not all preach the same messages, nor did members of the congregation receive the messages in the same ways.[59] The Heath family of Brookline illustrates such variances. Mary Heath chronicled her struggle with a debilitating condition in diary entries from 1824: "I began to feel very sick—so sick that I could hardly endure the sound of the fish which has [been] frying for Pa's supper or the laughing & playing of Abby & Sophia." She retreated to her "cold dreary chamber" and took simple remedies of "warm water, brandy & sugar, but found but little relief."[60] Mary found comfort in her religious beliefs. When she was able, she attended Brookline's First Congregational Church, the pulpit of Unitarian John Pierce. When Mary was incapable of attending services, she often read sermons. For example, on November 7, 1824, she enthused over the printed sermons of Dr. William Ellery Channing: "Miss Greene brought us Dr. Channing's sermons to read & such a sermon as it is so much piety, so much exalted sense, wisdom and feeling as is comprised in that sermon, I want to see the good Dr. more than ever."[61]

When Mary could attend church, she recorded her reactions to some of the sermons, allowing us a glimpse of how she viewed God's role in her illness. On November 21, 1824, Mary wrote what Mr. Pierce preached: "he told us how we should be affected by affliction that trials of this kind should tend to improve us, and prepare us for a better world than this."[62] Whether Pierce meant that God had sent Mary adversity as an opportunity to improve herself for salvation is less relevant than how Mary perceived the message. On July 27, 1824, she wrote:

> Father of mercies! Thou hast taught me by sickness to realize the vanity & uncertainty of the world. Thou hast shown me how frail I am—hath given me a striking proof of the precariousness of life. . . . May I be prepared for that illness from which I shall not recover—I thank thee for every comfort & alleviation of pain which thou hast been pleased to furnish me—I thank thee that thy powerful arm has arrested the progress of the destroyer—That at this season thou art permitting the cheering [word unreadable] health to revisit me.[63]

Mary Heath did not write of cures but sought relief through the medicine provided by Dr. Charles Wild, an orthodox physician. She did not experiment with several practitioners with different treatments. Her health was in God's hands; it was God who permitted health to visit or leave her. Yet she belonged to a Unitarian church.[64]

An explanation for this discrepancy may reside in how John Pierce handled internal church affairs at the beginning of the Congregational debate. Historian James McGovern states that Pierce attempted to remain neutral in the division between the Unitarians and the orthodox Calvinists in the early-nineteenth-century Congregational Church.[65] Thus, the Reverend Pierce may have provided a religious environment that allowed both traditional and liberal Congregationalists to worship under the same roof. Another explanation could be the nature of Mary Heath's condition. She suffered from a chronic condition that ultimately claimed her life at the early age of twenty. Those who suffered from debilitating illnesses, especially in their terminal stages, may very well have dismissed liberal tenets that did not serve them well and retained those traditional ideologies, such as God's special providences, that brought them comfort. Mary Heath serves as a reminder that religious beliefs, specifically special providences, did not exist strictly along denominational lines.

To complicate matters further, among Unitarians there arose a group of intellectuals who forged another spiritual path. Transcendentalism both sprang from and influenced Unitarianism. Some Unitarians such as Daniel Child and Lucy Chase sympathized with the radical beliefs of transcendentalism, while others did not. Although scholars do not share a consensus on exactly when transcendentalism began, by the end of 1836 participants were meeting in one another's homes, attending lectures, and reviewing works produced within their group. Transcendentalists agreed with Unitarians on several issues, such as Christ's lack of divinity and salvation through human agency. However, many Unitarians feared transcendentalists' rhetoric regarding the living God that resided in every person's soul, anxious that it bred agnostic tendencies.[66]

Early transcendental beliefs can be found in the words of Ralph Waldo Emerson. Just as Channing served as the unofficial icon of Unitarianism, Emerson became one of the major spokespersons for transcendentalism. He outlined his views succinctly in his famous Harvard Divinity School Address of 1838, wherein he refuted orthodox Congregationalists' views that man entered the world depraved. In Emerson's mind, man was born good and perfect and had to seek actively not to become evil and weak. There existed within each person an "intuition of the moral sentiment" that served as individual insight into "the perfection of the laws of the soul." Man had the divine intuition within himself, and as long as he did not distance himself too much from this intuition by committing misdeeds, he would be spiritually and physically healthy. "By it [the intuition of the moral sentiment] man is made the Providence to himself," and, as such, "he who does a good deed is instantly ennobled" and "he who does a mean deed is by the action itself contracted." How a man conducts himself determines what kind of life he has, and thus, by his own actions, he commits himself to heaven or hell.[67] When a man got "wide from God every year," he did so by "divine nature being forgotten, [whereby] a sickness infects and dwarfs the constitution." Man, according to Emerson, is born whole, but once he moves away from his own moral intuition (usually through materialism), he moves away from the divine. Yet, the "indwelling Supreme Spirit cannot wholly be got rid of," and so man suffers. Thus, both spiritual and physical illness can be seen as a perversion in which a person's constitution deteriorates through the struggle between what is divine within him and the suffering he has brought upon himself.

Boston transcendentalist Theodore Parker agreed.[68] He advanced, in his *Sermons on Theism, Atheism, and Popular Theology* (1853), a similar view of the primacy of human agency. Parker believed that the doctrine of Providence was dangerous because "man absolved himself from social responsibility by arguing that God controlled all according to His good purposes." He argued that social (and physical) ills "were a result of man's inactivity or mismanagement, not God's providence."[69] Thus, transcendentalists believed that sickness often arose from man's actions, and if a cure could be found, it would be through man's actions.

Caroline Dall provides an example of one transcendentalist managing family health care. Brought up as a Unitarian, she attended lectures by Emerson at the age of twelve and became a protégée of noted transcendentalists Elizabeth Peabody and Margaret Fuller.[70] In 1844, Dall married a Unitarian preacher. Through the years, she "strived to accommodate the new doctrines of Transcendentalism to her religious beliefs."[71] After the death of her son, she developed a friendship and long correspondence with Theodore Parker. Her beliefs are reflected in her journal. On March

24, 1850, she wrote: "We have had no health since we first came to Roxbury—partly I suspect because we have been pent up in one room." She did not attribute the series of illnesses that struck her family to God. She contracted influenza and a violent earache, which she treated ineffectively with blisters, blue pills, and warm baths. After experimenting with different remedies, she finally found relief through the application of leeches.[72]

When Dall's husband became ill, she relocated him to a better environment rather than praying to God for his recovery. She recorded: "I saw immediately that there was no time to be lost—and that whatever was the consequence to children still delicate with scarlet fever, the rooms must be changed. In less than an hour, I had him safely in bed below stairs. He seemed refreshed by the well ventilated pleasant room. 'It ought to cure me,' he said."[73] She had confidence in her own ability to act and to cure.

Although Dall did not record using homeopathic remedies, they attracted many transcendentalists.[74] Fuller argues that "homeopaths seemed to insinuate a more mystical view in which matter, if not exactly an expression of spirit, was at least receptive to spiritual infusions. For this reason, their healing system was avidly investigated by many followers of Transcendentalism."[75] Transcendentalists believed that some truths could not be obtained through intellectual reason (or sensory perception) alone, that an inner intuitive reason was needed. Thus, they were attracted to homeopathy, because its cure rested on infinitesimal doses to assist the body's vital spirit in overcoming disease, the effectiveness of which had been proven, if not explained, through experimentation (or "proving"). Homeopathy and transcendentalism shared the belief that some truths could not always be explained by the senses; some truths transcended reason.[76]

The famous Alcott family serves as a good example of transcendentalists' medical choices after homeopathy became more popular in Boston. When Elisabeth Alcott became ill in 1857, her father, A. Bronson Alcott, wrote to his other daughters to let them know how she was faring under the medical care of Dr. Christian F. Geist, a homeopathic physician in Boston: "Dr. Gheist [*sic*] has done much for her since he took her under his kindly care, and continues to promise of healing the dear patient in the reasonable time . . . her symptoms are less and less alarming, her sufferings being all mitigated by his prescriptions."[77] Although the Alcotts may have favored homeopathy, they often explored other medical treatments.[78] A. Bronson Alcott became a strong advocate for the water cure. Bronson held multiple lectures, or what he called conversations, on medical topics at Dr. Russell Trall's Water Cure Institute in New York; he even considered investing in one of Dr. Trall's institutes in 1856. Louisa May Alcott explored such medical options as magnetic therapy, botanical treatments, and the Mind Cure through the 1870s and 1880s, demonstrating her active search for cure among the latest remedies.[79]

Both Alcotts, however, often expressed doubt. In 1850, for example, Bronson contracted smallpox and corresponded with a relative that he "had a good appetite all the time, and kept the doctor out of the house, and so got well without medicines of any kind." Louisa confessed to a friend her use of magnetic therapy: "I'm going with Dr. L[awrence] to see Dr. Henion the magnetic man. A quack I dare say, but he cures people & the regulars don't, so for fun I'm going some day. Don't tell *any one* & I'll report." Louisa may have been skeptical of the efficacy of magnetism, but she was excited about the Mind Cure, in which a practitioner guided patients through meditation to reach the deep recesses of their minds and thus avail themselves of their divine healing energy. In realizing their oneness with "Infinite Life," patients such as Louisa could cure their disease themselves. She wrote to a friend that she had not been well and that she had "been trying the Mind Cure," and she found "it very wonderful. It is the power of the mind over matter, soul over body, & those who learn it can not only heal themselves but others, & live above the small pains & worries that vex so many of us." Eventually, though, Louisa became frustrated. "'It is,' they say, 'simply turning to the Source of all rest & strength &, sitting passive, let it flow into one & heal & cheer body & soul.' A very sweet doctrine if one can only *do it*. I cant yet, but try it out of interest in the new application of the old truth & religion which we all believe, that soul is greater than body, & being so should rule."[80]

Louisa and A. Bronson often expressed skepticism about medical treatments, but the Alcotts did investigate those medical applications that coincided with the "old truth & religion which we all believe"—namely, transcendentalism. Thus, the Alcott family searched among those medical treatments that dovetailed with the idea that both spiritual and physical health could be achieved through nature—whether through water, magnetic forces, mind over matter, the spirituality of homeopathic remedies, or botanical medicines. Transcendentalists believed that God had given man all he needed to be spiritually and physically at peace; if ill, it was up to each individual to renew health from within. They remained confident that cure as an eradication of disease was possible.

As Congregationalists in New England contended with the rise of Unitarians (and subsequently transcendentalists), they also entered into debate with evangelicals, whose ideas appealed to people across all denominations. Evangelicals' belief in providential acts gained renewed popularity in nineteenth-century Massachusetts with a Second Great Awakening that swept through the United States from the 1800s through the 1830s, in part as a response to the rationalization of religious doctrines among the traditional denominations—Congregationalists, Presbyterians, and Episcopalians. The first wave occurred on the eastern seaboard under the guidance of Timothy Dwight at Yale University. The tone of New England revivals differed from their western counterparts; New Englanders engaged in religious reform from pulpits rather than tent revivals and encouraged decorum rather than emotional displays. Under Lyman Beecher, Nathaniel Taylor, and Asahel Nettleton, the revival in New England remained within the walls of the brick-and-mortar church.[81]

The second wave of revivalism in New England began in 1831 when Beecher and others invited Charles Finney, a key figure in the Second Great Awakening, to Boston. From 1824 to 1827, he led a series of revivals throughout upstate New York, fueling another phase of religious intensity that spread to New England.[82] Finney made it clear in his *Lectures on Revivals of Religion* (1835) that humans must actively pursue conversion and then God would confer grace.[83] The Second Great Awakening represented conservative theological forces, but with common people playing a central role in their own salvation.[84]

Both Boston Unitarians and orthodox Calvinists condemned Finney's brand of revivalism. His theology aligned more readily with the that of the orthodox Calvinists; both believed in the divinity of Christ, his death and resurrection, and the need for conversion. However, the Second Great Awakening departed from traditional Calvinism, fusing evangelical theology with the theological position that emphasized free will in conversion. Revivalism centered on spiritual action to promote individual and societal reform. Beecher understood social reform in many ways as a traditional Congregationalist would: if a community ignored its sins then God would wreak havoc. But Beecher, like other revivalists, gave the message a more modern interpretation: the community that did not repent would suffer increased vice, which would destroy God's universal moral order and thus the community. Beecher's God would not send locusts; He would not have to. This explains why churches that participated in the Second Great Awakening encouraged social activism among their ranks. Revivalists became leaders in the antislavery and temperance movements as well as health reforms in order to combat vice.[85]

The revivalists' views on God's role in illness require careful consideration. On the one hand, they believed in free will and, on the other, in special providences through which God spoke to the depravity of man. As Finney preached: "The Spirit of God, by the truth, influences the sinner to change, and in this sense is the efficient cause of change. But the sinner actually changes, and is therefore himself, in the proper sense, the author of change." The Spirit of God does not give power to man, man has already been created with the power to obey Him; man has free will. The Spirit helps man "overcome his voluntary obstinacy." Illness, then, can be seen as one of God's "instruments he uses to change the sinner's heart." Finney criticized traditional Congregationalists, who appeared "to be passive, to wait for some mysterious influence, like an electric shock, to change their hearts." Thus, patients who participated in revival viewed illness as part of God's plan, an opportunity for sinners to overcome their "voluntary obstinacy," and yet were urged to be active in the pursuit of medical treatment.[86] Health, like salvation, was a gift from God, but man had to choose to accept the gift. After all, God helped those who helped themselves; but evangelicals across denominations believed that God's help was needed to recover from illness—more so than denominations featuring stronger threads of rationalism.

Julia Cowles of Farmington, Connecticut, offers an example of early revivalists' attitudes toward illness. She attended the services of Timothy Dwight and sought medical care from Dr. Eli Todd.[87] Cowles's diary contains her belief in God's actions in illness. On April 15, 1802, she wrote concerning her father's return to health: "It [illness] teaches us our dependence on God.... Every day we see enough to convince us that of ourselves we can do nothing, that it is God who works in us to will and to do, that it is of his sovereign grace and mercy that we are yet spared, are this side [of the] grave, while many are cut down and sent to a long and eternal home."[88] Like Fiske, Cowles saw illness as God's work. She viewed sickness and injury as an opportunity either to prepare one's self spiritually or, if spared, to recognize God's mercy firsthand. Illness became a learning opportunity for all who suffered or witnessed it.[89]

Sophronia Grout of Hawley, Massachusetts, represents an ideal revivalist, both demographically and spiritually. According to one historian, young unmarried females who worked in textile factories or as schoolteachers comprised the largest demographic group of those reborn. As the daughter of the Reverend Jonathan Grout of the First Congregational Church, unmarried, and a teacher, Sophronia outwardly appears to have been a typical evangelical of her time. Contemporary preachers repeatedly commented that "the converted were neither self-assertive nor self-righteous—they expressed humility, and continued in self-doubt. Conversion came not as a lightning bolt, but as a gradual struggle.... they had to report that the best subjects for conversions were young persons who had been reared in families of some piety."[90] Demonstrating a similarly gradual struggle with piety, Sophronia recorded on July 14, 1816: "My evidence of change of heart is but small very small indeed.... What evidence have I of any saving change?"[91] Sophronia was reared in piety, yet she agonized over the veracity of her conversion, mirroring the ideal spiritual posture of a revivalist.

Bemoaning her inability to pursue the evangelical commitment to social reform or even to attend religious meetings, Sophronia often struggled with what role she would play in "benefiting fellow creatures." Her poor health meant that she could not participate in social activism or useful labor, as she was often bedridden. She studied to improve herself but wondered how such study benefited others. On March 2, 1825, she prayed: "Heavenly Father will thou direct me in the way of duty—Let me not be a vile, useless worm." Likewise, she recorded that she could not participate in religious services on May 1 and prayed that "God of heaven would make me a lowly humble Christian he would make me acquiesce cheerfully in every dispensation of his Providence."[92]

When Sophronia did attend her father's church, he gave firm guidance on how to respond to struggles. Adversity is the hand of God, "who has laid this rod upon you." "And however severe the smart," the Reverend Grout exhorted his congregation to remember that "He chastens for your profit. ... If any of you are unacquainted with God, you may find it to be good for you to be afflicted. It shows you your dependence on God, the evil effects of sin, the importance of reformation of the heart and life."[93] Sophronia heeded her father's words. She believed herself to be more religious due to her illness: "I wish not to forget the seasons of affliction. . . . I have learnt from this affliction which I could not have gained from the best Divines in the world. Those who are the most acquainted with human nature could not by the most artful reasoning have convinced & instilled into my mind so deeply as experience has done. I would often review those days of darkness, They were not in vain."[94] Sophronia understood her illness to be God's will. She sought His guidance on how to reform herself as well as society through her illness.

Yet the Grout sisters were not passive about their diseases. Sophronia's sister Esther also struggled with illness as an evangelical. Esther sought relief from the hot springs of Saratoga Springs, New York, in 1830. In June, she complained that she was not receiving as much relief as she had the previous year and bemoaned the fact that she did not have any time in which to "pour out my soul in prayer to God" because she feared she would be disturbed; in this case, medical treatment interfered with her ability to pray. However, her visit to Saratoga did provide her an opportunity to pursue the evangelical mission of societal reform, for Esther found herself among the unsaved. On several occasions she records that she spoke to the Browne sisters about the state of their souls. One of the Brownes was not appreciative: "She did not appear to feel so grateful to me for speaking to her upon the subject of religion as did her sister."[95] Some pursuits of better health precluded privacy for prayer, but they did provide opportunities to convert, however reluctant the audience.

Esther took several trips to visit a sister in Hamilton, New York, to benefit her health. She decided that a change in climate might be favorable to her lungs. Unfortunately, her active pursuit of healthier climes did not help. On February 16, 1834, she penned that she had "commenced spitting blood again." She faced a conundrum as she treated herself. On the one hand, when she treated her lungs, it aggravated her other ailments. On the other, when she took remedies for her other ailments it would "injure" her lungs. "I never so needed the services of a skillful physician as at present," Esther wrote. Interestingly, neither Sophronia nor Esther regularly mentioned medical treatments. Esther spoke of her physician several times, but never mentioned his name or the treatments he prescribed. Both dedicated their journals to understanding God's purpose for them, especially as invalids, rather than any pursuit of cure.[96]

While the physician or physicians who treated the Grout sisters cannot be discerned from their journals, some supposition is possible. At the time they kept their journals, the community of Hawley could boast of having one physician, Moses Smith.[97] Described by one historian of Hawley as an "orthodox physician who long practiced in town," Smith practiced regular medicine from 1810 until his death in 1849.[98] It appears that the Grout sisters were treated by regular doctors. Of course, this may have been a function of the limited choices in rural areas. Yet Esther did not appear to notice the lack of medical choices. "Since I came home I have seen none [doctors]." Although she had taken a turn for the worse on February 16, 1834, she wrote that she knew of "no better way for me to do than be content with my situation and trust in the Lord. He can heal me without the aid of earthly physicians or He can sanctify my present afflictions to my soul and prepare me for a peaceful and happy death."[99] She understood the outcome of illness ultimately to be in the hands of the Great Physician and that any earthly physician could only provide guidance in relief, not cure.

Although both Cowles and the Grout sisters may have chosen orthodox physicians, scholars have made connections between revivalists and unorthodox medicine. Historian Robert C. Fuller argues that revivalists or the unchurched were more drawn to it. Revivalists may have been drawn to Thomsonian practitioners because of shared ideologies. Thomsonians encouraged people to make use of God's natural laws to assume responsibility for their own physiological health with a faith in human perfectibility similar to that which evangelical preachers displayed when they urged their followers to assume responsibility for their own salvation. In fact, Fuller asserts that "Thomsonianism spread along precisely the same geographical lines that revivalist preachers traveled (i.e., roughly from Vermont and New Hampshire into western New York State and into the Ohio Valley) spreading the new theological mood of optimism and perfectionism."

Of the revivalists' diaries I have found, few demonstrate a strong connection to Thomsonian medicine. Of the three analyzed here, Cowles's diary predates Samuel Thomson's rise to medical fame, and the Grout sisters could have utilized the Thomsonian system—Esther did reveal that she self-medicated—but they never recorded doing so.[100] What Cowles's and the Grouts' diaries do show is that conversion did not mean complacency. Revivalists reformed and labored for salvation; it was God's gift. Likewise, they sought and labored for good health; but, ultimately, life was God's gift to give or take. They could not rest assured of good health any more than they could rest in certainty of salvation.

Unitarians, Congregationalists, transcendentalists, and revivalists understood God's role in illness differently, but these religious categories do not serve as distinct demarcations as to how each believer would respond to illness. By the 1840s, the differences between Congregationalists and Unitarians had begun to blur, while revivalists could be found among all denominations, making sharp distinctions between members of different denominations difficult. Two elements appear to have predicted patients' expectations and responses: belief in special providences and whether a patient was a reforming or radical member of her/his denomination. For example, Child and Chase, as Unitarians sympathetic to transcendentalism and active reformists, illustrate Unitarians who experimented with all types of scientific medical treatments. Conservative Unitarians such as Louisa's husband, John Park, did not. Park described transcendentalism as "chiefly a disconnected series of vague dogmas," which reflects his rejection of the more radical transcendentalism.[101] The Parkses did expect to find a cure in the more modern meaning of the word, but they expected to find it in more traditional medical practice (after all, John Park himself was a regular practitioner). The Grout sisters, as revivalists, understood God's role in a traditional way but still sought treatment at spas, demonstrating that, conservative or radical, most nineteenth-century believers actively pursued an understanding of God's natural laws and took action to live in harmony with them. Where they differed was on the point of God's direct or indirect guidance in understanding natural laws (including illness) and how to find harmony (and health) in the natural world.[102]

Changes in religious beliefs did not mean a lack of piety. For decades patients understood heroic medicine to be helpful in providing relief—if not cure—from various ailments. This was understandable in light of their religious beliefs. Afflictions came from God, and only through Him would they find cure; physicians could provide relief through small mercies. However, as the nineteenth century progressed, patients who held certain religious beliefs sought (and believed they could find) cure in various medical treatments. Many scholars describe changes in popular ideas of pain and illness as a "process of secularization," describing unorthodox medical systems as "fraught with notions of metaphysical causality that ran counter to the general tide of secularization."[103] But viewing the metaphysical as counter to secularization seems inadequate. Patients, such as Fiske, challenged this dualistic conception of patients' religiousness and view of science by demonstrating that a patient could be an educated, rational, and savvy consumer of medicines while still believing that illness was part of the metaphysical.[104] Also, an individual could be religious and yet be open to trying newer scientific treatments, like the Childs family. An extreme example are the followers of Sylvester Graham's health-reform movement, who engaged in a scientific pursuit of health that constituted a religion.[105] Transcendentalists sought health in nature as a way to reconnect with their moral intuitiveness, their link to God, and thus their cure. Catherine Albanese's model of three Christian points of reference—God, humanity, and nature—whose emphasis shifts into a spectrum of spirituality, seems more fitting than to see the nineteenth century as a process of secularization. Influenced by their religious beliefs, each of the individuals discussed here determined how God, humanity, and nature interacted. Patients' understanding of the roles each of these forces played in illness influenced their medical choices and their interpretations of the meaning of cure, as well as their expectations of finding it.

5

Medicine and Malpractice

In the May 29, 1844, issue of the *Boston Medical and Surgical Journal* (*BMSJ*), an article appeared outlining the malpractice trials of a Dr. Colby of Vermont. The author dramatically sympathized with Colby's fate: "He had been tortured under the legal screws nearly as much as a man can bear—his case having been protracted year to year, and from court to court."[1]

Suing a physician for malpractice is the epitome of unmet patient expectations. Mid-nineteenth-century patients increasingly understood cure as the total eradication of disease and held medical practitioners to a higher standard of care than they had previously. As patient expectations changed and industrial accidents multiplied, the law as applied to medical care evolved from seeing malpractice as akin to nuisance to viewing it as negligence. The intersecting of patient expectations, cultural changes (religious and economic), and a medico-legal evolution resulted in a surge of malpractice cases by the mid-nineteenth century.

From the 1850s onward, more and more physicians like Dr. Colby found themselves in court. Historian Kenneth DeVille reported that of the 216 appellate malpractice decisions he analyzed throughout nineteenth-century America, only 5 occurred before 1835.[2] In contrast, state supreme courts ruled on 42 malpractice cases between 1835 and 1870, 45 cases from 1870 to 1880, and 47 cases from 1880 to 1890, outpacing the increase in population.[3] This increase in malpractice suits levied against doctors has been attributed to a wide variety of factors, including the breakdown of community mechanisms to resolve disputes, a preoccupation with health, and an emerging view of the body as mechanical.

In Massachusetts malpractice suits rose around the 1850s as well. From my analysis of thirty-one cases between 1847 and 1873 in lower and appellate courts other influences and motivations emerged.[4] Certainly, the demise of local mechanisms for conflict resolution and depictions of bodies as mechanical contributed to an increase in malpractice cases. But these address only the plaintiff's view. A fuller understanding of the surge in medical malpractice suits has to include a confluence of attitude changes among all the participants in the trials—judges, juries, physicians, and patients. In bringing suits, patients (plaintiffs) became active negotiators for their own health care in conversation with multiple parties who had different interests.

Malpractice cases began with dissatisfaction with medical care and/or cost of care. Most physicians and patients worked out their differences without having to resort to law suits. Frequently, disputes between doctors and patients involved fees. Physicians' daybooks contain many entries involving "reckonings" or adjustments to amounts owed because patients believed they had been overcharged. For example, Moses Mosman of Sudbury recorded in 1771 that he "reckoned balance and settled all accompts with Mr. Ephraim Goodenow and rec'd by a note of hand in full"; or, as he did in 1805, Mosman recorded a conversation with Mr. Conant in which he wrote "rec'd by your account and by a note in full"—Mosman had adjusted Conant's debt after discussion and then received a note from him on the adjusted amount.[5]

Occasionally physicians and patients could not resolve their disputes over charges and quality of care themselves, especially if permanent bodily or financial damage had been done. In these instances, patients could sue for medical malpractice. American malpractice law emerged from English common law. The term "malpractice" derives from the Latin *mala praxis* (bad practice). In the widely referenced *Commentaries on the Laws of England* (1768) Sir William Blackstone defined it as "Injuries, affecting a man's *health,* are where by any unwholesome practices of another a man sustains any apparent damage in his vigour or constitution. As by selling him bad provisions or wine; by the exercise of a noisome trade, which infects the air of the neighborhood; or by the neglect or unskillful management of [a patient's] physician, surgeon, or apothecary . . . because it breaks the trust which the party had placed in his physician, and tends to the patient's destruction." Significantly, Blackstone compared medical practice to trades, such as those which might be "noisome" and disturb the neighborhood, or those which might sell tainted food or spirits. As he discussed it, medical malpractice fell under a category of law akin to nuisance. In these cases, plaintiffs needed to prove that a physician's actions had robbed a patient of the use of his body.

In the eighteenth century, medical malpractice was not considered a broken contract but a personal wrong. As patients sought help from physicians voluntarily, strictly speaking the writ of trespass did not apply, because it applied to damages resulting from direct force to a person or his property. Blackstone allowed for remedy in damages by an action of "trespass, upon the case," which would serve as a universal remedy for all personal wrongs and injuries without the exertion of direct force. English common law held that physicians' liability and responsibility for patients did not derive from a commercial contract but from "the affirmative act of entering into the doctor–patient relationship."[6] A physician's responsibility lay in his understood role as a community healer who professed to have an expertise, not by terms outlined in a written document. Although elements of negligence can be found in Blackstone's discussion, eighteenth-century malpractice focused on injury, not failure to perform.[7]

Courts saw few legal actions brought against physicians in the eighteenth century. Prior to the American Revolution, most disputes (malpractice among them) found resolution within the community, where town meetings, churches, and courts shared responsibility for mediating conflicts. Towns dealt with disputes between groups of people concerning issues such as road placement, use of streams, and public health. Courts overwhelmingly dealt with debts. One historian estimates that 74 percent of the civil suits heard by justices of the peace in Plymouth County, Massachusetts, concerned debts. Churches exercised their authority over individuals guilty of fornication, breaches of the Sabbath, and drunkenness. In Plymouth County, "juries and congregations both decided disputes in accordance with similar normative standards," thus often having overlapping duties.[8]

By 1820, an increase in all types of litigation had occurred in Massachusetts. The increase in litigation in Plymouth County, for example, was not just a function of commerce and population but, some have argued, indicated a breakdown of informal mechanisms of dispute resolution. In particular, given the importance of local congregations in community resolutions, the increase in religious pluralism fostered greater divisions among local populations, making the resolution of disputes by the church less effective. People who had always been litigious turned more and more to the courts.[9]

Before 1830, professional journals such as the *BMSJ* provided little commentary on malpractice. Nor did any treatises on the subject exist. As general litigation rose, physicians began to serve as medical witnesses in court cases. Thus, most medicolegal texts focused on medical jurisprudence (the application of medical knowledge to legal matters), not malpractice issues. In the nineteenth century, Theodric Romeyn Beck advised many elite American physicians on how to be effective medical witnesses in his *Elements of Medical Jurisprudence* (1823), which covered topics such as the role of physicians in determining fitness for military service, paternity, rape, insanity, and murder, especially poisonings.[10]

Medical jurisprudence offered an opportunity to practitioners who were willing to testify in court cases, bolstering their public image as members of a respected profession. As one historian described it, "the physician who solved a public mystery, rid his community of toxic pollution, identified a dangerous murderer, or saved an innocent local citizen from wrongful conviction became a public hero." In one Pennsylvania case that gained notoriety, three physicians' testimonies helped to convict John Earls of poisoning his wife's tea with arsenic after she had given birth to a child. Presumably, Earls had hoped that his wife's death would look like the result of childbed fever. Unfortunately for him, however, the county coroner asked three physicians to conduct a postmortem in which doctors ran tests that showed a large amount of arsenic present in the remains. The contents of Catharine Earls's stomach were sent to experts at the Medical Institute at Philadelphia, who performed more tests. In May 1836, John Earls was hanged for his crime. The story of his trial, published as a book and circulated nationally, proved the value of professional medical expertise in trials.[11]

John J. Elwell's *A Medico-Legal Treatise on Malpractice, Medical Evidence, and Insanity, Compromising Elements of Medical Jurisprudence* (1860) became one of the first American publications to deal substantially with malpractice. Contemporaries recognized this treatise as the authority on legal standards of care to which physicians were held. Quoting Nicholas C. Tindal, chief justice of the Court of Common Pleas in England from 1829 to 1846, Elwell outlined the doctrine of common law that applied to the professions of medicine and law: "every person who enters into a learned profession, undertakes to bring to the exercise of it a reasonable, fair and competent degree of skill."[12]

Elwell's standard for physicians represented a shift in the legal notion of malpractice that developed over the course of the nineteenth century. In the early decades, the dominant understanding of malpractice involved negligence, a physician's failure to fully perform the duty imposed by an implied contract between doctor and patient. Now, the issue was not just whether or not an injury had occurred, but what had caused the injury.[13] This was no small matter to determine. The rule of reasonable skill applied to physicians carried various exceptions. *McCandless v. McWha* (1853) provides a clear demonstration of legal standards for malpractice and its exceptions.

James McWha of Pennsylvania claimed that Dr. Alexander G. McCandless caused him "an injury sustained by reason of alleged Malpractice, in the setting and treatment of his broken limb. This action was brought to September Term, 1848." The jury awarded damages of $850 to McWha. McCandless appealed the case in the Pennsylvania Supreme Court in 1853. The basis of the appeal rested on the claim that the judge had erred in his jury instructions. The Supreme Court agreed, reversed judgment, and granted a new trial.[14]

Jurists often cited *McCandless v. McWha* in medical malpractice cases. In Judge Woodward's majority opinion the lower-court judge had instructed the jury: "That the defendant [the physician] was bound to bring to his aid the skill necessary for a surgeon to set the leg . . . and if he did not, he was accountable for damages, just as a stonemason or bricklayer would be in building a wall of poor materials, and the wall fell down." The Pennsylvania Supreme Court ruled that this was an impossible standard for a surgeon to uphold. Although the same standard of ordinary care was applied to tradesmen, the standard differed in each profession. In other words, as defined by the Pennsylvania Supreme Court, ordinary care meant the care exercised by those practicing the same trade. Furthermore, Elwell explained, "the implied contract of a physician or surgeon is not a cure—but to treat the case with diligence and skill." Discrepancies between popular meanings of cure as the eradication of disease or ailment and the professional understanding of cure as treatment became most obvious in malpractice cases.[15]

Physicians and surgeons did not perform the same kinds of tasks as a stonemason or bricklayer, the court ruled. McWha's fracture was seen as more complicated to repair than brick and mortar. The patient "may, by willful disregard of the surgeon's directions, impair the effect of the best-conceived measures," whereas a bricklayer did not give homeowners any directions that would impinge on the result of his work. In other words, the shortening of McWha's leg might have resulted from "the most careful and approved practice, or from the misconduct of the patient."[16] In other words, the doctor could not control whether or not a patient followed his directions. This reflects the emerging role played by contributory negligence in American law.[17]

Malpractice claims in nonsurgical treatments proved even more difficult to establish. As Elwell shows, mitigating circumstances arose in every medical case, especially nonsurgical treatments. He offered several categories of examples, including "debilitating factors" (improper nourishment or care by family, impure air, intemperance); "accidental or acquired predisposing causes" (earlier bouts of malaria, infections, or previous injuries); "congenital conditions" (epilepsy, stunted growth, and circumstances of age); "hereditary conditions" (gender, inherited debilities); and "temperament" (melancholy, nervousness, or irritability). Therefore, a physician or a surgeon could not predict the outcome of cases due to factors over which he had no control. Here lay the difference between medical practice and science; in medicine there existed "a want of that uniformity so beautiful and remarkable in other branches of physical science."[18] Medicine did not have the luxury of the controlled environment available in laboratories.

In a lengthy *Boston Medical and Surgical Journal* article, Suffolk County lawyer Alexander Young attempted to explain malpractice law to physicians, acknowledging that patients levied charges of malpractice against surgeons more often than against other physicians. "The process of surgical art is more palpable than the operations of the physician, and the results of treatment are more obvious in the former case than in the latter. . . . The surgeon is too often regarded as only a skillful mechanic." He argued that the scientific knowledge of how to treat surgical cases was much easier to convey than "the scientific knowledge which determines the necessity of an operation," the latter being a more "valuable attainment in a surgeon."[19] Similarly to the modern claim that a patient does not pay an anesthesiologist to put him to sleep but to wake him up, the nineteenth-century surgeon's valuable expertise did not lie in the know-how of a surgery but in knowing when a surgery was necessary. Young attempted to explain to his physician-readers that patients oversimplified the practice of medicine, which led to unmet expectations and malpractice suits.

The difficulty in receiving damages for medical malpractice due to the variety of exceptions can be demonstrated by a review of *Hibbard v. Thompson* (1872). In this malpractice case in the latter decades of the nineteenth century the modern notion of negligence becomes more evident. Emery Hibbard claimed that Dr. Augustine Thompson of Lowell began treating him for rheumatism or rheumatic fever on March 11, 1871. Hibbard claimed that Thompson had ceased to attend to him on April 5, and subsequently he developed a bedsore. The sore became so painful that on April 10 Hibbard "was obliged to go to the hospital and remained there for a month, and for a long time [this] kept" him from his occupation as a blacksmith. The defendant countered that the plaintiff did not suffer from a bedsore but from a wound. Hibbard had fallen on the bed rail, and the sore was the result of neglect of the wound by Hibbard and his home-based caretakers. The jury found for the defendant doctor. Hibbard filed for appeal on exceptions, because the judge had refused to instruct the jury that this was not a case "where the doctrine of contributory negligence" applied. The Supreme Court overruled the exceptions, claiming that there was sufficient evidence of contributory negligence. As Elwell had observed, the doctor rarely controlled external factors, including the safety of the patient's environment. Because of the array of external factors that might exist to mitigate the physician's responsibility, patients who sued for malpractice had a difficult time proving it, especially in medical as opposed to surgical cases.

This is one explanation of why, as Elwell claimed, "nine-tenths of the medical malpractice suits arose from either treatments of amputations, dislocations, or fractures." In 1860, a physician studied 142 cases of malpractice and found that almost two-thirds of them involved orthopedic procedures, 102 of them fractures and 32 stemming from dislocations.[20] Out of the 31 Massachusetts cases between 1847 and 1873 that I have identified, 19 involved orthopedic procedures such as amputation, bone setting, and treatment of dislocation of a joint (see appendix C). Prior to the 1870s, many nineteenth-century malpractice cases appear to have involved surgery mishaps regardless of which region of the United States was studied.

Conant v. Manning (1849) demonstrates the difficulties that patients had collecting damages in surgical cases. For example, Francis Conant of Stow, Massachusetts, fell under an ox-drawn carriage while bringing a load of wood to Lunenburg on December 27, 1847, fracturing his jaw and dislocating his thigh bone. Dr. Peter Manning of Lunenburg was called in and attempted to reduce the dislocation, but had a hard time keeping the bone in place due to a fracture of the hip socket. After resting for several weeks as instructed, Conant returned to Stow against Manning's advice. On March 2, he returned to Lunenburg to see Manning, at which time Conant claimed his leg was better and he no longer needed to wear the belt Manning had prescribed to stabilize the leg. On March 22, at the advice of his family physician in Stow, Conant sought care in Massachusetts General Hospital (MGH) where he underwent an operation to improve the limb. As a result, one of Conant's legs was two inches shorter than the other.

Conant sued Dr. Manning, claiming that he had misrepresented the condition of his leg and thus caused damage. In the first trial, several MGH surgeons testified on behalf of the defendant, stating that it was a hard case and that there was no indication that Dr. Manning lacked skill or had demonstrated want of care. Nevertheless, the jury came back with damages of $362.50. Manning demanded a new trial on the grounds that the verdict went against trial evidence. The judge agreed and set aside the verdict, ordering a new trial. A new trial ended in the jury awarding Conant damages of $100.00. Again the verdict was set aside by the bench, at which point the case was dropped.[21]

As *Conant v. Manning* shows, a plaintiff might find it easy to sue and even be awarded damages by a jury, but collecting those damages was difficult. Although juries often awarded damages to plaintiffs, in Massachusetts the judges in many instances set aside the verdict. In this case, the judge did so twice because the evidence seemed to reveal two issues: (1) Conant did not follow Manning's orders, either by staying in Lunenburg to allow his hip to heal completely or by wearing the belt that stabilized his leg for the full amount of time prescribed by Manning; and (2) the testimonies of noted MGH surgeons who stated that Manning had employed the necessary skills in his care of Conant. The court did not hold Manning to the standard of total cure in such a complicated case as dislocation of the femur and a fractured hip socket. However, the plaintiff as well as the jury did.

Scholars and contemporaries alike have discussed the attitudes and motives of plaintiffs. Orthodox physicians regularly attributed the bringing of malpractice suits to poor patients who were trying to avoid paying their medical debts or to turn an unfortunate medical outcome into a hefty payout. In one journal the author summarized *Edgely v. Bartlett* (1854), a case in which one physician was forced to spend a lot of time and money to defend his professional reputation. Dr. Bartlett had to withstand three trials; two with no verdict reached by the jury and the third with a verdict for the defendant. "The defendant came off victorious, and the plaintiff remains, as at the beginning, without a shilling drawn from Dr. Bartlett's pocket," the author declared with satisfaction. But Bartlett defended his character and reputation with "heavy expense."[22] Plaintiffs often shouldered the high cost of multiple trials over long periods of time. If plaintiffs were hoping for a substantial payday, then malpractice suits represented an unwise gamble given that many trials reported in the medical literature (and reprinted in newspapers) resulted in verdicts in favor of the defendant/physician. Even verdicts against physicians were often set aside.[23]

One report of *Rice v. Thorndike* (1855)—another case decided in favor of the defendant after two trials—argued that if plaintiffs such as Rice were awarded damages of $5,000 for the loss of a toe from well-respected physicians such as William H. Thorndike of Boston, then legal changes would be necessary to protect the medical profession.[24] Indeed, at the appellate level, cases showed that plaintiffs disproportionally sued the best, well-respected physicians such as Dr. Thorndike. In attempting to explain this, one scholar offers several reasons, including the fact that "patients had little or no incentive to sue marginal healers with few assets, but substantial incentive to sue the most prosperous physicians, from whom they might actually collect."[25] However, the conclusion that most malpractice cases involved impoverished patients suing wealthy doctors is problematic. A systematic survey of appellate cases does show that a disproportionate number of well-to-do physicians were sued, but a systematic survey of cases at the trial-court level has not been made. One could imagine that cases pursued to the appellate level rather than being dropped might have been perceived as more winnable. The Massachusetts cases studied here do not reveal any propensity to sue the best of physicians. Certainly, physicians such as Henry L. Sabin, a trustee of the State Lunatic Hospital at Northampton, held positions of note, but Ira Perry of Medway did not.

Plaintiffs were not necessarily poor either. In the thirty-one malpractice cases analyzed, twenty-seven plaintiffs' names were given and eighteen occupations of plaintiffs could be identified (see table 5.1). Only a few could be categorized as impoverished: a peddler, a farmer (although one farmer's real estate was valued at $3,500 by the federal government), a worker in boot factory, and a domestic. In these cases, the plaintiffs could not be accurately described as impoverished patients suing well-to-do physicians in search of a large payoff. After all, physicians had been treating impoverished patients long before the surge in malpractice cases occurred.[26] The increase in plaintiffs willing to sue their physicians came from a growing sector of industrial workers and tradespeople.

Both skilled and semiskilled workers sued in Massachusetts. Most of them shared occupations with those who entered the MGH discussed in chapter 3. They belonged to the categories of industrial workers and traditional tradesmen—gunsmith, master harness maker, shoe finisher, cigar maker, baggage master, boat builder, ship carpenter, blacksmith. This group of people comprised an aspiring population, one not just interested in escaping poverty but in acquiring some wealth or property—until illness or injury occurred. For example, orthopedic disabilities could lead to a sudden, marked decline in lifestyle for a skilled or semiskilled worker. Unlike the impoverished, these workers had an economic footing to lose, and they lost it suddenly through their disability. This constituted a financial setback they could not afford as the upper classes could.

Medical malpractice charges leveled by skilled and semiskilled workers fit into a broader legal trend. Legal historian Morton Horwitz argues that the gradual decay of a paternalistic relationship between workers and employers caused an increase in the number of employees who sued their employers for injuries resulting from negligence. Before 1840, workers' injuries "were probably compensated out of benevolence or charity, depending on the extent of personal relationship between master and servant." With the advent of railroads, the risk of serious injury of employees rose alongside a breakdown of paternalistic behavior on the part of employers. Thus, more and more laborers turned to courts seeking compensation. At the same time, judges often set aside verdicts in railroad cases because "juries took into account speculative factors that if allowed would hinder commercial development or be deemed unfavorable to the community as a whole."[27] Judges pondered the impact of verdicts on the whole society, not just on each individual.

Many of the underlying causes in the rise of industrial tort cases explain the surge in malpractice suits. Patient–physician relations shifted in ways similar to employer–employee relations. Prior to the mid-nineteenth century, physicians had operated and were perceived as community healers, often demonstrating benevolence. As physicians came to be seen more as commercial actors, the personal reciprocal obligation between patient and physician (in both economic and social terms) declined. This shift, as I argued in chapter 3, altered the medical experiences and expectations of middle- and working-class people in different ways. Skilled and semiskilled workers were the most negatively affected. Perhaps, then, it should not be surprising to find that in the thirty-one cases studied here, many plaintiffs were skilled and semiskilled workers.

Juries often viewed matters in much the same way as plaintiffs did. Attitudes among jurymen arose from their public perceptions of medical practitioners. Printed media influenced those perceptions.[28] Ironically, physicians, in their attempts to professionalize medical practice, authored books that also contributed to public views of the human body and the profession of medicine among plaintiffs and juries. Many nineteenth-century popular books and lecture series informed the public on topics such as health, hygiene, and the body. True, maintaining health was not a new topic and medical advice books existed prior to the nineteenth century. However, up until the mid-nineteenth century these texts did not include lengthy passages on anatomy and physiology. Nonphysicians began to spark public interest in anatomy and physiology as keys to better hygiene and health.

For instance, William A. Alcott found much success with his series of essays "The House I Live In," published as installments in magazines in 1833. Alcott focused on human anatomy, often linking domesticity, hygiene reform, and Christian morality to the body. By doing so, he urged the public to involve themselves in preserving their health as a moral as well as physical imperative. He carried the analogy of the construction of a house with that of the body throughout the text, beginning with chapter 1, "The Framework of the House: The Thigh Bone. The Leg, etc.,"[29] thus implying that a body could be as easily understood by readers as the frame of a house could.

Many educated physicians sought to exploit the hygienic reform movement in print to popularize science and to elevate themselves as participants in it. As the Earls case demonstrated, physicians testified as court experts on a range of medical and scientific matters, which were reported in newspapers and, in sensational cases like Earls's, in books. But as orthodox physicians identified themselves more and more as professionals and scientists, they came under increasing accusations of being elitist. In the 1830s, Jacksonian Democrats abhorred monopolies and opposed professional licensure. Competing medical sects opportunistically adopted the free-market, common-man rhetoric and used it to undermine orthodox, educated regulars. In an attempt to bridge the gap between the educated elite and the common man, physician-authors sought to reconnect with their patients through creating health treatises.[30]

Described by one historian as the greatest influences on popular understandings of anatomy and physiology, Massachusetts physicians Calvin Cutter, Edward Jarvis, and Thomas Lambert wrote books in the 1840s that explained the human body in mechanical terms. For example, Cutter's *The Physiological Family Physician, designed for Families and Individuals* (1845), along with other of his works, "were fabulously successful, going into multiple stereotyped and revised editions, and were translated into Tamil, Arabic, Japanese, Russian, and other languages."[31] Cutter often used common analogies to make the inner workings of the human body more accessible to his readers. For example, he described the joints as being "constantly supplied with a fluid called syn-o'-vi-a," which "operates like oil on the joints of a machine." Muscles and tendons are to the bones, he stated, "what the ropes are to the sails and yards of a ship. By their action, the direction of the sails and yards is changed. So, by the action of the muscles, the position of the bones of the body is changed." Cutter made religious remarks throughout his text, as did Alcott. He reminded his readers that they should "be lost in wonder" when "contemplating this superb and intricate machine, formed and finished by the Great Architect."[32] These writers equated understanding anatomy with understanding God's gifts. Jarvis added to the public understanding of physiology with his *Primary Physiology, for Schools* (1848), in which he described heart valves as having the same purpose as "the valve of a pump-box, which opens to let water pass upward, but closes and prevents its passage downward."[33] Cutter and Jarvis made anatomy and physiology more accessible by drawing these analogies to everyday mechanical objects.

In a similar fashion, Lambert showed equal talent in explaining the human body. Dr. J. D. Mansfield reviewed Lambert's *Popular Anatomy and Physiology* in an 1850 issue of the *BMSJ*. He speculated that "there was nothing, in my opinion, that would so soon and so completely rid the community of charlatanism, as a good knowledge of some of the first principles of medical science." For this reason, Mansfield recommended Lambert's text to any general reader who wished "to keep up with the intelligence of the time."[34] Many such editorials in the *BMSJ* applauded the attempts to educate the public about anatomy, physiology, and hygiene through texts and lectures in the hope that such efforts would create an informed public who could appreciate the difficulties of medical practice. But some editorials revealed the downside of attempts to popularize medical knowledge. The public had become more informed, but, as one physician lamented in 1848, "the truth is, it [the public anatomy lecture] is a superficial show of superficial things, and far too often [delivered] by very superficial persons in pursuit of pence."[35] The analogies used in popular texts did produce a more informed public, but it also reinforced an expectation that the physician should be held to the same standard of performance as any tradesman.

Given the mechanical analogies provided by popular anatomy and physiological books for general readers, it is little wonder that in cases like *McWha v. McCandless* the jury (and even lower-court judges in this case) expected to have physicians, especially surgeons, fix broken legs as a carpenter would fix a broken spindle on a chair. *Conant v. Manning* demonstrates equally well that the public as exemplified by a jury continued to hold physicians to standards similar to those they expected from many tradesmen.[36]

As malpractice cases were reported in newspapers, further challenges to the image of the medical profession arose. These cases often underscored the conflicting opinions that occurred among medical practitioners. Medical jurisprudence may have created medical heroes in some instances, but conflicting testimonies in malpractice cases publicized the absence of widespread agreement on medical care. What hurt regular physicians the most, however, was not competition between them and other medical sects, but disputes among themselves. Nowhere did the absence of unity in the medical profession become more apparent than in the courtroom.

In the Massachusetts malpractice case *Ashworth v. Kittridge* (1853), a ten-year-old boy had had his left hand mangled "in a picker of [a] woolen mill." The boy suffered severe wounds and a simple fracture to the radius. The boy's father, John Ashworth, claimed that his son's arm had to be amputated because Dr. Joseph Kittridge of North Andover had provided improper care. At the trial, a veritable war of medical opinion ensued. Dr. I. D. Pilsbury of Lowell testified that the bandages applied by Kittridge were too tight, cutting off the boy's circulation from the lower arm. He also stated that the bandages were not checked frequently enough by Kittridge, who did not realize that gangrene had set in until the fourth day. Drs. George Hayward, S. D. Townsend, Frederick Ainsworth, and H. L. Bigelow of Boston testified for the defendant, claiming that proper care had been given, and that if the bandages had been tight enough to cut off circulation, then the pain would have been intolerable, leading to patient complaints about it. They also testified that a tight bandage would not cause gangrene; the plugging of the artery would. The jury heard an array of medical opinions and finally awarded the plaintiff $1,675.[37]

Unfortunately for the medical profession, conflicting medical testimonies did not remain within the courtroom. Several notices about *Ashworth v. Kittridge* appeared in newspapers, and the case was discussed in professional journals, as were other cases with conflicting medical testimonies. Physicians well understood the harm of such public displays of medical disunity. In *Edgely v. Somerville*, Emma Edgely sued a Massachusetts physician for not reducing her fractured clavicle, resulting in her having only partial use of her right arm. One author describing the case in a professional journal wrote that "it is whispered about in judicial circles that the testimony of the experts in surgery, who were called in, was contradictory to a more than usual degree. Some of them gave an unqualified opinion that the collar bone had never been broken. Others advanced other views; and on summing up the whole, it would have puzzled a Philadelphia lawyer to discover from it what had been the matter."[38] If professional identity relied on demonstrating good medical practice, then open debates in court over just what constituted good medical practice undermined the process of building such professional identity. Jurymen's (and future jurymen's) perceptions of the medical profession would have been influenced by such reported conflicts among medical experts.

In cases in which juries concluded that malpractice had occurred and plaintiffs deserved compensation, judges did not always agree. Among appellate cases across the country identified by DeVille, physicians prevailed in "well over half the malpractice suits of 1835–1865."[39] Newspapers and professional journals remarked on the frequency of judges ruling against jury verdicts. One paper in 1856 reported that six malpractice cases had been tried in Middlesex County, Massachusetts, in the past six years and that "four verdicts were returned; and all, after careful examination were set aside by the whole court, showing that the jury must have been mistaken in the evidence, or were influenced in their decisions by prejudice."[40]

Changes in the roles of judges also influenced outcomes. Before the nineteenth century, jurists had viewed common law and legislative statutes as distinct bodies of law. Conceived as a fixed, customary body of legal doctrine, common law was derived from natural law, and a judge's role was to apply it to individual cases. Over the course of the late eighteenth and early nineteenth centuries, American legal theorists began to justify common law by consent rather than expressing it in terms of custom derived from natural law.[41] The shift resulted in more verdicts being set aside.

Judges' tendency to set aside verdicts in medical malpractice suits can be compared with a broader change seen in industrial tort cases such as the landmark case of *Farwell v. Boston and Worcester R.R.* (1842). A railroad engineer, Nicholas Farwell, drove over a track that had been improperly left open by a switchman. The train derailed, and Farwell, thrown from the train, had his hand crushed by its wheels. Customary principles held a master liable for tortious acts of his servants, including any negligence resulting in injury to a servant performing his duties. As in this case both the injured engineer and the switchman worked for the same employer, the court could choose to follow the fellow-servant rule. The rule (simply put) stipulated that a servant or employee who was injured by the actions of a fellow servant or employee could not claim damages from the master or employer. Farwell argued that the fellow-servant rule did not apply in this case because he and the switchman were not fellow servants but were hired to do distinctly different jobs, and thus were not jointly employed for a common purpose.[42]

The presence of railroads after 1830 meant an increase in worker injuries like Farwell's. In this case, as in others, the competing claims about the legal relationship between employer and employee become evident. In *Farwell v. Boston and Worcester R.R.*, Chief Justice Lemuel Shaw of the Massachusetts State Supreme Court relied on a more contractual idea of the relationship between employer and employee. Legal scholars have argued that Shaw and other jurists understood wages to be a carefully negotiated tool "by which supposedly equal parties would bargain to arrive at a proper 'mix' of risk and wages." In other words, by accepting wages, Farwell also accepted the risks of injury inherent in the performance of his job. *Farwell v. Boston and Worcester R.R.* highlights the move toward a doctrine of "assumption of risk" in workmen's injury cases and, as such, shows the shift toward an understanding of the employer–employee relationship as contractual.[43] Such opinions favored legal outcomes that promoted economic growth (in this case, the building of railroads) over individual interests.[44]

As it came to be conceived of as a product of consent and will, judges began to consider common law as equally important as legislation for promoting social policies. Verdicts no longer involved outcomes only of individual cases but of public policy.[45] For instance, in medical malpractice, too many verdicts requiring that large damages be paid by surgeons would inhibit surgical practice and prove detrimental to society as a whole. As malpractice suits became more common, physicians threatened to refuse treatment in surgical cases or to demand that patients unknown to them sign waivers. The *BMSJ* reported that Dr. Josiah Crosby of New Hampshire refused to treat a fractured limb "unless the patient would place himself under bonds not to prosecute in the event the limb should not be perfect." The author advised that this was the only safe course for surgeons to take, because "the rage to obtain money from surgeons in unsuccessful cases is only paralleled by the suits against railroad companies."[46] Contemporary physicians understood malpractice suits as falling within the broader phenomenon of increasing negligence suits, as did judges. If juries were allowed to continue to award heavy damages to plaintiffs, then industrial expansion would be curtailed, and there would be no surgeons or physicians willing to treat workers injured in the rising number of industrial accidents.

One of the most important consequences of a shift in legal conceptions of common law and the role of the judge was the change in the relationship between judge and jury. Before the nineteenth century, juries had held a vast amount of power to determine both the law and the facts of cases. Although several devices existed in English common law to control jury findings, few were employed in Massachusetts before the nineteenth century. Between 1805 and 1810, Massachusetts judges increasingly assumed powers formerly held by the jury. For instance, judges routinely began to determine the law and instruct the jury as to the laws that applied to the case. If a judge believed that a jury's verdict went contrary to the facts of the case, then the verdict would be set aside.[47] These changes in conceptions of common law and judicial authority explain why many of the malpractice cases in Massachusetts, such as *Conant v. Manning,* saw jury verdicts set aside.

When deaths occurred, malpractice suits could be brought to criminal courts. In Massachusetts, charges against physicians for murder or manslaughter due to malpractice appeared early in the nineteenth century but were rare. *Commonwealth v. Thomson* (1809), a charge of murder leveled at Samuel Thomson, father of the Thomasonian botanic system of medicine, became an oft-cited case in later malpractice suits. Thomson stood trial in Salem for the death of Ezra Lovett. Allegedly, he had treated Lovett over the course of several days, giving him multiple large doses of an emetic. Many witnesses testified to having observed the patient's great distress. When Thomson asked Lovett how far the medicine had gone down, the deceased laid his hand upon his breast, to which Thomson responded that "the medicine would soon get down and *unscrew his navel*"; this was interpreted to mean that the medicine would soon reach Lovett's intestines and have a cathartic effect. Instead, he went into convulsions, while Thomson continued to dose the patient with emetic powders. The convulsions continued until Lovett died.

Chief Justice Theophilus Parsons of the State Supreme Judicial Court told the jury that if there was no proof of malice, either expressed or implied, then they could not return a verdict of guilty on the charge of murder. Although the solicitor general in the case argued that Thomson was guilty of manslaughter because "he rashly and presumptuously administered to the deceased a deleterious medicine, which in his hands, by reason of gross ignorance, became a deadly poison," the bench instructed the jury that if they believed Thomson had acted with an *honest intention* to cure by this treatment, and death was merely an unexpected result, then he was not guilty of manslaughter. After the jury applied the judge's legal standard to the facts of the case, it reached a verdict of not guilty.[48] Parson's instructions became the standard for decades to come.

By the late nineteenth century, a more rigorous standard emerged for criminal prosecution of malpractice than the one set forth by the Thomson case. Eventually, lack of training or skill did not excuse a practitioner from criminal liability if improper treatment resulted in death.[49] As with most criminal liability, criminal malpractice required proof of malicious intent. Although providing positive evidence was often difficult, circumstantial evidence could be established. If it could be shown that a physician, based on his knowledge or means of knowledge, should have known his treatments were unsafe, then an implication of malicious intent could be made. Physicians by entering their vocation assumed a responsibility for treatments and remedies that could be dangerous. By the later decades of the nineteenth century, if a physician abused such treatments, whether through ignorance, negligence, or malice, causing death, then he could be charged with manslaughter or murder.[50] In other words, had Thomson been tried in the mid-nineteenth century, he would likely have been found guilty.

As the law regarding criminal malpractice evolved, more cases emerged in Massachusetts, including suits against nonregular practitioners. Inquests, coroner's juries, and other legal announcements in Massachusetts newspapers give us glimpses of these cases. Some announcements offered few details, such as one involving Dr. Hill of Boston, charged with the death of a domestic. The victim's name was not clear, nor were any details regarding the specifics of the cause of death. Other items gave more details, such as the reported findings of a jury of inquest in the *Springfield Republican*. Professor William W. Greene of Berkshire Medical College underwent examination in the death of Adilla Jones of Lee. Greene had treated Jones for chronic uterine disease. The newspaper reported that, after six days of deliberation and "a vast amount of evidence . . . some of which was very conflicting," the jury returned the following verdict: "That said Adilla H. Jones died at Pittsfield, on Friday night April 6, 1866, and the immediate cause of death was intense inflammation of the stomach and bowels, termed enteritis, which was produced by the severe treatment of Dr. William Warren Greene at his office, on the 31st day of March, A.D. 1866, and by his neglect to give proper care after said treatment."

Issues in the case show the transmission of contributory negligence to the educated populace since *Commonwealth v. Thomson*: the coroner's jury did not excuse Greene even though he demonstrated honest intentions. While four jurors returned a verdict of negligence, two, George P. Briggs and George Gay, dissented. Briggs believed that there was no direct connection between treatment and the inflammation that caused Jones's death. He stated that the "nervous shock" due to the treatment and her predisposition in "connection with exposure to cold and dampness and rain" had caused the inflammation.[51] Here, Briggs articulated the contributory negligence detailed in Elwell's 1860 treatise and that was raised in courtrooms from the 1860s on.

Reports of criminal malpractice appeared in newspapers involving other medical practitioners as well. Abortionists, midwives, physicians, and others—all were brought to criminal court on charges of murder and manslaughter by the 1860s.[52] Midwife Mrs. Goodwin was charged with manslaughter. After delivering the baby of Mrs. Samuel Breckenridge, Goodwin mistook an inverted uterus for a tumor and cut it out. Breckenridge bled to death shortly after the physician arrived. But as one jurist remarked, determining when negligence became egregious enough to be proof of malice was not easy: "Between willful mischief and gross negligence ... the boundary line is hard to trace. ... [T]he law runs them into each other."

In U.S. malpractice cases (both civil and criminal), legal handbooks and various jury and court rulings underscored the ambiguous legal standing of death and injury by malpractice, suggesting "that the law was beginning to reflect the contractual aspects of the doctor–patient relationship as well as the legal duties associated with a common calling."[53] The law tended to blur the distinction between tort and contract in malpractice cases, and because it did, outcomes of such trials varied (see appendix C). Not until after the Civil War did the modern understanding of negligence (in which carelessness becomes the central allegation) become distinct.[54]

Another difficulty arose in distinguishing patient–physician relationships as community-based or contract-based in origin. Here lies a confluence of factors that shifted patient expectations of medical services, wherein patients began to see physicians as "individual entrepreneurs in an intensely competitive marketplace." As discussed in chapter 3, doctors and patients increasingly engaged in separate cash transactions rather than in reciprocal, long-term exchanges that involved mutual trust as well as obligation.[55]

In sum, plaintiffs experienced a change in their relationships with their physicians due to shifts in several cultural factors, and patients' expectations of medical care rose in the nineteenth century among both rich and poor. Newspaper advertisements bombarded readers (and possible future plaintiffs) with promises of cure—cure defined as total eradication of disease or restoration to an able body. Changes in religious beliefs fostered a different understanding of how God worked through illness and injury. To be ill or permanently injured was no longer automatically equated with God's punishment or considered a trial of faith. Instead, disease was seen as a result of mankind's own actions, one that could be corrected if health—both moral and physical—was pursued correctly. If patient expectations were not met, patients no longer depended on community conflict-resolution mechanisms and increasingly turned to the law courts for redress. Patient-plaintiffs pursuing malpractice suits tended to be members of an aspiring industrial group in Massachusetts, skilled and semiskilled workers whose very livelihoods were threatened by illness and injury. No longer resigned solely to submit to God's will, they became much more likely to blame their physicians and to actively seek compensation.

But exploring plaintiff-patients motives does not reveal the whole story. Changes occurring among all the actors must be explored in order to understand why malpractice suits in the early part of the nineteenth century were virtually nonexistent only to surge after 1840. Jury verdicts reflected public interpretations of patient–physician relations that had transitioned from community-based reciprocal interactions to more contractual ones. Physicians attempted to establish themselves as participants in science and professionals with medical expertise. They became medical witnesses in court. Some wrote treatises to foster a greater public understanding of physiology and anatomy and to underscore the complexities of their expertise. In doing so, they raised patients' expectations of their services, sometimes in ways not intended. Plaintiffs and juries often conflated their expectations of tradesmen's work with that of a physician. Yet judges saw malpractice cases in a broader context. Their responsibilities expanded to include applying laws to individual cases, often with the public's best interests in mind rather than those of individual parties. This, along with the emerging idea of contributory negligence, resulted in many jury verdicts in favor of the plaintiff being set aside.

Malpractice suits became a microcosm of legal negotiations between parties with different economic goals and expectations for medical care. Patient expectations heightened over the course of the nineteenth century and became consistent with the rise of negligence as the basis of malpractice law. Thus, it was transformations in cultural factors—economic and religious—alongside legal changes that fostered an environment in which judges, juries, plaintiffs, and physicians increasingly met in court to continue to negotiate the burdens of disease and disability.

Conclusion

The history of medicine is most often recounted from the viewpoint of the medical profession, even though that tells only half of the story; for patients also shape medical practice through the choices they do or do not make, and that was no less true of nineteenth-century patients than it is of patients today. As the subtitle of this book suggests, societal changes in economics, religion, and law all affect patients' attitudes toward medical care, and those attitudes in turn determine whether and how they decide to be treated.

In the nineteenth century, physicians saw themselves as scientists. However, treating the human body created by the Great Architect entailed so many variations that their profession proved to be an inexact art. Medical practitioners strove to implement the newest strategies and theories of their profession but always had to keep in mind that "patient curing" (as physician Worthington Hooker described it) had to be balanced with "patient getting." In other words, physicians needed to be responsive to their patients' expectations if they wanted a thriving practice. Doctors offered more than a commercial service. They probed into patients' most intimate bodily functions (a departure from stereotypical private and prudish Victorian mores) and entered private homes as observers of family dynamics.

Both the commercial and the intimate aspects of medical practice gave rise to several difficulties. In economic matters, local exchange systems that did not measure success by mere profit allowed for payment in many forms, resulting in complex webs of credit and debt that appear to have mirrored the complexities of the patient–physician relationship. In the 1820s economic exchange systems in urban areas began to alter, and the long-distance trade system that gradually emerged required regular, if not immediate, payments in cash or promissory notes. The rise in physicians' insistence on being paid in cash or notes demonstrated an increasing financial insecurity. Yet physicians found it a delicate matter to insist on immediate payment. How could one maintain a close professional relationship with one's patients while demanding cash or notes in times of illness?

Those who possessed cash or social credit would become active medical consumers who shopped for cures, not simply as treatments for relief, but to eradicate disease. Beginning in the 1820s, the impetus for an increase in alternative medical practitioners such as homeopaths and water curers came from changing expectations of medical care rather than long-held dissatisfaction with medical therapeutics. Regular physicians responded to those expectations, espousing a theoretical framework for a more conservative therapeutic approach, one that many Massachusetts physicians were already using.

Changing expectations did not derive from economic shifts alone. As reformers within various denominations broke away from the traditional Congregationalism that had dominated the Massachusetts religious landscape, they challenged traditional medical practice. No longer content with enduring illness passively, they did not wait to be spiritually saved or physically healed. Unitarians, for example, held high hopes for the fruits of scientific research to eradicate disease, though not at the expense of their piety. There were congregants who believed that God had given man the will to act—religious activism fed patient activism.

Any medical care that resulted in further injury or death increasingly led to the filing of malpractice suits in the hearings of which the court was obliged to evaluate the relationship between patient and doctor. In legal terms, the patient–physician relationship proved difficult to categorize, fitting neither the laws pertaining to contracts nor the laws covering personal injury. Malpractice cases reflected the confusion over the exact nature of the medical relationship in the new commercial, industrialized world of the early American Republic. The law also reacted to the shifts in medical relations in the context of surging industrial accidents and an increasingly mobile population. Courts moved from judging malpractice cases under the legal rubric of nuisance to one of negligence, with contributory negligence becoming more common in judicial opinions by the late nineteenth century. Thus, we see a confluence of societal factors changing patients' expectations of their health care, reshaping demands for medical therapeutics by the mid-nineteenth century.

Medical relationships underwent another transformation between the late nineteenth and early twentieth centuries. Beginning in the late nineteenth century, the medical profession became more cohesive, confident, and self-congratulatory. Doctors celebrated current medical practice based on scientific discovery as far superior to the brutal depletive heroic therapies of yesteryear. With the advent of germ theory at the end of the nineteenth century and the rise of institutional care (to name only two influencing factors), physicians' confidence in their profession grew, and many historians of medicine pinpoint a change in the medical relationship, often describing it from the medical profession's point of view or characterizing it as increasingly physician-dominated.[1]

Paul Starr describes the shift in medical relations that occurred between the 1870s and 1900s as one marked by a widening social distance between practitioners and patients due to the consolidation of professional authority by doctors. Factors such as the growth in the American Medical Association's membership through collaboration with other medical competitors, particularly homeopaths and eclectics, opened up access to financial and political resources that allowed the AMA to push for licensing, the reform of medical education, and the oversight of patent medicines. In this discussion, Starr describes the "public's increased reliance on professional opinion in decisions about medication."[2]

Was the public indeed more reliant on physicians' opinions about therapeutics? Starr thinks so, locating the growth in authority (which he defines as a "surrender of private judgment") in various developments, such as muckraking journalism that exposed the dangers of nostrum makers and their potions, which made medical consumers more wary.[3] Key scientific discoveries and innovations in diagnostic technology added to the professional standing of physicians. One crucial development occurred in the 1860s and 1870s with the work of French chemist Louis Pasteur and German physician Robert Koch in bacteriology. A result of their discoveries was that, by the 1890s, public-health measures taken against infectious diseases improved health on a public scale, especially by controlling water-borne (sand filtration of the water supplying lowered instances of typhoid) and food-borne (regulation of milk supplies decreasing infant mortality) diseases. The first major therapeutic application of bacteriology occurred with the development of a diphtheria antitoxin in the mid-1890s. Alongside developments in science, new diagnostic techniques strengthened the authority of practitioners and radically altered the doctor–patient relationship. The stethoscope, the microscope, and the X-ray, among other instruments, provided medical information that did not require patients' subjective input. Simultaneously, these innovations inspired a greater confidence in the authority of medicine.[4]

More recently, Nancy Tomes has underscored the significance of the discovery of germs and how awareness of them changed notions of disease and became "part of the fabric of everyday life."[5] As she correctly points out, the first fifty years after the acceptance of germ theory, most of the emphasis was placed on the prevention of disease through modification of individual and public hygienic behavior. She explores the collective consciousness in the understanding of germs and disease during this watershed moment in medical history.[6]

While many pages have been dedicated to the individual scientists, experimental discoveries, and institutional responses to germs and changing views of infection, Tomes provides a study about the domestication of germs. A wonderful addition to this literature would be to explore the consequences of the rise in the modern view of infection and use of diagnostic technology for patient expectations and the medical relationship. I suspect that physicians' new scientific knowledge did contribute to a relationship in which patients deferred to physicians' expertise in certain matters, but not in any systematic way. The doctor's authority most likely held sway in certain areas of treatment such as that for tuberculosis. It seems plausible that in common ailments such as constipation and pain relief treatments remained part of the patient's purview.

This book has tried to contribute to the first part of the traditional narrative from 1790 to 1860 by looking at medical therapeutics through patients' eyes. As the brief discussion above demonstrates, the period from the 1860s to the 1930s presents another opportunity to reexamine medical history through tracing patient expectations and experiences during an important era of transition. But that is another book for another time.

TABLES

Table 1.1. Moses Mosman, Sudbury, MA, 1786–1793

INGREDIENT/PROCEDURE (*most common use*)	TIMES PRESCRIBED	PERCENTAGE OF 537 TOTAL
Lavender	47	9
Proprietatis, elixir (stomachic)	44	8
Camphor (narcotic)	31	6
Asthmaticus, elixir (narcotic)	29	5
Dressing	27	5
Volatile salts (antispasmodic)	26	5
Cathartic, not specified	21	4
Delivery	15	3
Emetic, not specified	14	3
Medicines, not specified	13	2
Bleeding	11	2

Source: Moses Mosman, Account book, 1763–1820, MSS, folio vol. "M," American Antiquarian Society, Worcester, MA.

Note: Only ingredients with greater than 1% usage are listed. Percentages have been rounded.

Table 1.2. Moses Mosman, Sudbury, MA, 1802–1820

INGREDIENT/PROCEDURE (*most common use*)	TIMES PRESCRIBED	PERCENTAGE OF 943 TOTAL
Camphor (narcotic)	109	12
Paregoric, elixir (narcotic)	72	8
Lavender (tonic)	57	6
Cathartic, not specified	52	6
Delivery	47	5
Proprietatis, elixir (stomachic)	46	5
Emetic, not specified	35	4
Niter, spirit of (cathartic)	29	3
Rhei (cathartic)	28	3
Medicines, not specified	27	3
Peru, cortex (tonic)	24	3
Bitters (tonic)	23	2
Vitae, balsam (tonic)	23	2
Bleeding	18	2
Epispastic, not specified	18	2
Spigelia [Marilandica] (anthelmintic)	16	2
Dressing	15	2

Source: Moses Mosman, Account books, 1763–1820, MSS, folio vol. "M," American Antiquarian Society, Worcester, MA.

Note: Only ingredients with greater than 1% usage are listed. Percentages have been rounded.

Table 1.3. Abraham Lowe, Ashburnham, MA, 1786–1798

INGREDIENT/PROCEDURE (*most common use*)	TIMES PRESCRIBED	PERCENTAGE OF 1,302 TOTAL
Paregoric, elixir (narcotic)	70	5
Tartar, emetic	54	4
Calomel (cathartic)	51	4
Camphor (narcotic)	51	4
Glauber's salt or vitriolated soda (cathartic)	46	4
Bleeding	42	3
Jalap (mild cathartic)	37	3
Dressing	36	3
Chamomile, florae (tonic)	32	2
China or Cinchona (tonic)	27	2
Emplastrum, epispastics (blistering plaster)	27	2
Specific Amara (stomachic)	27	2
Surgery, minor and bone setting	26	2
Pulled tooth	26	2
Valerian, radix (antispasmodic)	24	2
Antimony, essence/powder/pill (cathartic)	21	2
Aurantium [hispalense] cortex (tonic)	21	2
Caryophyllum rubrum (flavoring)	21	2

Source: Abraham Lowe, Medical account book (photostat), 1786–98, N-2084 (oversize), Massachusetts Historical Society, Boston, MA.

Note: Only ingredients with greater than 1% usage are listed. Percentages have been rounded.

Table 1.4. William Stoddard Williams, Deerfield, MA, September 1786–February 1791

INGREDIENT/PROCEDURE (*most common use*)	TIMES PRESCRIBED	PERCENTAGE OF 320 TOTAL
Dressing	30	9
No medicine	23	7
Calomel (cathartic)	17	5
Bleeding	15	5
Rhei (mild cathartic)	14	4
Catharticus sal or vitriolated soda (cathartic)	12	4
Caryophyllum rubrum or Dianthus (flavoring, sometimes cardiac or alexipharmic)	11	3
Pulled tooth	11	3
Febrifuge, unspecified	11	3
Emetics, unspecified	9	3
Aeithiops mineralis (anthelmintic)	8	2
Turner's Cerate (unguent)	8	2
Sulphur, flowers of (cooling cathartic)	7	2
Stomachicum, elixir or Stoughton's Bitters (tonic)	6	2
Ammoniac[us], sal (diaphoretic)	5	2
Cream of tartar (mild cathartic)	5	2
Emplastrum, epispastic (blistering plaster)	5	2
Jalap (cathartic)	5	2
Magnesia (antacid)	5	2
Valerian, radix (antispasmodic)	5	2

Source: William Stoddard Williams, Daybook, September 1786–February 12, 1791, vol. 1, PVMA no. 13185, Pocumtuck Valley Memorial Association, Deerfield, MA (PVMA).

Note: Percentages have been rounded. Each ingredient charged to a patient's account under a specific date was counted as an entry. See Table 1.11 for list of ingredients used less than 1%.

Table 1.5. William Stoddard Williams, Deerfield, MA, June 1804–March 1806

INGREDIENT/PROCEDURE (*most common use*)	TIMES PRESCRIBED	PERCENTAGE OF 446 TOTAL
Cream of tartar (mild cathartic)	34	8
Cathartic, not specified	25	6
Jalap (cathartic)	23	5
Thebaica, tincture (opium)	17	4
Calomel (cathartic)	16	4
Tartari, Sal (diuretic)	15	3
Anodyne (opium)	14	3
Emetic, not specified	14	3
Rhei (mild cathartic)	14	3
No med	13	3
Dressing	13	3
Saturn, extract of, or cerussa acetate (astringent)	10	2
Pulled tooth	10	2
Chamomile, florae (tonic)	9	2
Emplastrum, diachylon	9	2
Tartar solution (mild cathartic)	9	2
Unknown	9	2
Bleeding	8	2
Plaster, unknown or not specified	8	2

Source: William Stoddard Williams, June 1804–March 1806, Daybook, vol. 24, PVMA no. 13185, PVMA.

Note: Percentages have been rounded. See Table 1.11 for list of ingredients used less than 1%.

Table 1.6. William Stoddard Williams, Deerfield, MA, June 1825–August 1828

INGREDIENT/PROCEDURE (*most common use*)	TIMES PRESCRIBED	PERCENTAGE OF 561 TOTAL
No medicine	39	7
Cream of tartar (mild cathartic)	37	7
Calomel (cathartic)	33	6
Cathartic, not specified	32	6
Thebaica, tinctura (opium)	23	4
Bleeding	21	4
Benedicta laxative (strong cathartic)	17	3
Jalap (cathartic)	17	3
Ricini, oil (mild cathartic)	17	3
Emetic, unspecified	15	3
Antimony, essence/powder/pill (cathartic)	15	3
Anodyne (opium)	14	3
Camphor (narcotic)	12	2
Lavender (tonic)	12	2
Opium (narcotic)	12	2
Colocynthis (violent cathartic)	12	2
Delivery	11	2
Emplastrum, epispastic (blistering plaster)	11	2
Scillae or Scilliticae Pilule (diuretic)	10	2
Pulled tooth	9	2

Source: William Stoddard Williams, June 25, 1825–August 12, 1828, Daybook, vol. 24, PVMA no. 13185, PVMA.

Note: Percentages have been rounded. See Table 1.11 for list of ingredients used less than 1%.

Table 1.7. Stephen West Williams, Deerfield, MA, July 1836–October 1838

INGREDIENT/PROCEDURE (*most common use*)	TIMES PRESCRIBED	PERCENTAGE OF 532 TOTAL
Dover's Powder (diaphoretic w/opium)	63	12
No medicine	48	9
Calomel (strong cathartic)	38	7
Cathartic, not specified	25	5
Jacobi (unknown)	19	4
Antidyspeptic, not specified	19	4
Chloric, ether (sedative?)	18	3
Paregoric, elixir (narcotic)	18	3
Bleeding	17	3
Hiera Picra (cathartic)	15	3
Rhei (mild cathartic)	13	2
Ricini, oil (cathartic)	12	2
Opium	11	2
Oxmel: scilli (diuretic)	11	2
Chinchona or quinine (tonic)	11	2

Source: Stephen West Williams, July 19, 1836–September 19, 1843, Daybook, vol. 24, PVMA no. 13185, PVMA.

Note: Only ingredients with greater than 1% usage are listed. Percentages have been rounded.

Table 1.8. Caleb H. Snow, Boston, MA, January 1827–December 1828

INGREDIENT/PROCEDURE (*most common use*)	TIMES PRESCRIBED	PERCENTAGE OF 543 TOTAL
No medicine	206	38
Opium (narcotic)	27	5
Calomel (strong cathartic)	23	4
Indecipherable	14	3
Antimony, essence/powder/pill (cathartic)	10	2
Camphor (narcotic)	9	2
Ipecac (emetic)	9	2
Rhei (mild cathartic)	9	2

Source: Caleb H. Snow, Account book, Caleb H. Snow Papers, 1775–1945, Massachusetts Historical Society, Boston.

Note: Only ingredients with greater than 1% usage are listed. Percentages have been rounded.

Table 1.9. Use of heroic therapeutics (percent)

PHYSICIAN	BLEEDING	CALOMEL	OTHER TYPES OF MERCURY	CATHARTIC	EMETIC	OPIATE/ NARCOTIC	NO MED.
Mosman 1786–1793[1]	2	0	0	17	3	12	.7
Lowe 1786–1798	3	4	1	25	5	13–14[2]	.6
William S. Williams 1786–1791	5	4	0	25	5	3	7
Mosman 1802–1820	2	1	0	20–21[3]	4–5[4]	20	1
William S. Williams 1804–1806	2	4	0	33	4	10	3
Snow 1827–1828	.7	4	1	14	2	10	38
William S. Williams 1825–1828	4	6	0	36	6	11–13[5]	7
Stephen Williams 1836–1838	3	7	0	23–24[6]	.5	22–25[7]	9

Notes:

1. Mosman kept two overlapping account books. I sorted the data in these two account books by dates and selected a comparable range to Lowe's and W. Williams's account books.
2. I express data as a range because six times Lowe prescribed a sedative (it was unclear if it was an opium) and six times prescribed saponaceous pills (soap pills made with either rhei or opium).
3. Range due to saponaceous pills (see note 2) and a dose-dependent drug, antimonii vitrum ceratum (either a cathartic or an emetic, depending on the dose).
4. See note 3 on antimonii vitrum ceratum.
5. Higher percentage occurs if one counts sedatives.
6. Range is due to antimonii vinum (either a cathartic or an emetic, depending on dose).
7. Higher percentage occurs if ether is added to the category.

Table 1.10. Types of cathartics used (percent)

PHYSICIAN	MEDS USED[1]	% OF USAGE	MILD[2]	MODERATE[3]	STRONG[4]	UNSPECIFIED
Mosman 1786–1793	18	17	7	3	3	4
Lowe 1786–1798	17	22	7	8	1	4
W. Williams 1786–1791	15	24	9	8	6	0
Mosman 1802–1820	17	17	7	3	2	6
W. Williams 1804–1806	14	33	19	3	4	6
Snow 1827–1828	17	12	5	1	6	0
W. Williams 1825–1828	12	31	15	1	9	6
S. Williams 1836–1838	10	23–25	6	4	9	5

Notes:

Percentages in the last four columns are those of total entries and may not add up to the total of percentages of cathartics used due to rounding.

1. Number (not a percentage) of different kinds of cathartics used, when specified.
2. J. Worth Estes, *Dictionary of Protopharmacology: Therapeutic Practices, 1700–1850* (Canton, MA: Science History Publications, 1990). Cathartics not specified are not included. Mild cathartics include rhei, ricini oil, cream of tartar, jalap, soda phosporata, Frankfurt pill, magnesia vitriolata, polychrestum balsam, sulphur balsam, liquorice or glycerrhiza, and a lenitive.
3. Moderate cathartics are those that work reliably but slowly and/or are given no description such as weak or strong. They include hiera picra, flowers of sulphur, sanguinaria Canadensis, hydragyrus pill, rufus' pill, salutis elixir, sambuccus (nigra), and sapo.
4. Strong cathartics include calomel, rhamnus catharticus, tigilii oleum, plummer's pill, magnesia alba, and senna.

Table 1.11. Ingredients and procedures used less than 1 percent by William Stoddard Williams

SEPTEMBER 1786–FEBRUARY 1791 INGREDIENT (*times prescribed*)	JUNE 1804–MARCH 1806 INGREDIENT (*times prescribed*)	JUNE 1825–AUGUST 1828 INGREDIENT (*times prescribed*)
Anodyne (1)	Absinthum, sal (1)	Althaea vitriol (1)
Ansi[e] (3)	Aethiops mineralis (4)	Amara (1)
Anthos, oil (1)	Alexipharmic, unspecified (1)	Ammoniaci, spiritus salis (1)
Antimony, essence/powder/pill (2)	Aloes (3)	Ammoniae acetatae aqua (2)
Arabic Gum (2)	Amara (3)	Ansium (1)
Asthmaticus elixir (3)	Ammoniaci, lac (1)	Antimonium tartarisatum or tartar emetic (1)
Camphor (1)	Ansi[e] (4)	Antimonium vitrificatum (1)
Camphor Gum (3)	Anti-icteric, not specified (3)	Armenian, bole (4)
Cantharis or cantharides (4)	Antimony, essence/powder/pill (7)	Asthmaticus, elixir (4)
Castor oil or oil ricini (3)	Arabic gum (1)	Aurantium [hispalense] cortex (1)
Caustic, not specified (1)	Armenian, bole (1)	Borax (6)
Chamomile, florae (4)	Astringent, not specified (1)	Catharticus sal or vitriolated soda (5)
Cicuta (1)	Borax (3)	Caustic, not specified (1)
Cinchona or Peruvian bark (1)	Camphor (3)	Cerate, not specified (1)
Cinnamon, cortex (1)	Camphor gum (1)	Chamomile, florae (8)
Cochiae, pilule (2)	Caryophyllum rubrum or Dianthus (2)	Cinchona or Peruvian bark or cortex (8)
Digitalis (1)	Castor[eum] (1)	Cinnamomum, cortex (2)
Dulcified spirits of niter (3)	Catharticus sal or vitriolated soda (5)	Copaiva (1)
Emplastrum, diachylon (1)	Cinchona or Peruvian bark (4)	Digitalis (2)
Emplastrum, roborans (1)	Cuminum (1)	Diurectic, unspecified (2)
Ferrum vitriolatum or sulphas ferri (1)	Digitalis (3)	Dressing (7)
Foetidae, pilule (1)	Dover's Powder (4)	Dulcified spirits of niter (5)
Foetidae, tincture (3)	Elemi, unguent (1)	Emmenagogues, unspecified
Glycerrhiza or glabra (1)	Emplastrum, epispastic (2)	Emplastrum, diachylon (2)
Guiaiac (2)	Emplastrum, oxycroceum (4)	Emplastrum, oxycroceum (1)
Hydragyrus muriatus corrosive (1)	Febrifuge, not specified (3)	Emplastrum, roborans (1)
Guiaiac (2)	Emplastrum, oxycroceum (4)	Emplastrum, oxycroceum (1)

Table 1.11. Ingredients and procedures (*continued*)

SEPTEMBER 1786–FEBRUARY 1791 INGREDIENT (*times prescribed*)	JUNE 1804–MARCH 1806 INGREDIENT (*times prescribed*)	JUNE 1825–AUGUST 1828 INGREDIENT (*times prescribed*)
Hydragyrus muriatus corrosive (1)	Febrifuge, not specified (3)	Emplastrum, roborans (1)
Indecipherable (2)	Foetidae, pilule (1)	Ether or aether vitriolicus (1)
Ipecac (2)	Gentian (1)	Eupatorium (3)
Lavender (3)	Glauber's Salt or vitriolated soda (1)	Febrifuge (3)
Magnesia alba (1)	Glycerrhiza or glabra (4)	Ferrum ammoniatum (1)
Manna gum (2)	Hydrargyrus muriatus corrosive (2)	Galanga (1)
Niter salt (1)	Indecipherable (6)	Gentian (1)
Niter, unknown (1)	Ipecac (2)	Glycerrhiza or glabra (4)
Plaster, not specified (3)	Julepum nuit? (1)	Indecipherable (4)
Oliva oil (1)	Lavender (4)	Ipecac (8)
Ophthamia, aqua (1)	Magnesia (4)	Jacobi, pulv. (1)
Potassae citratis, liquor (4)	Magnesia alba (1)	Laxative, unspecified (1)
Sacra, tincture (2)	Marini, spiritus salis (2)	Magnesia alba (1)
Saturn, extract of, or cerussa acetata (2)	Mentha piperita or peppermint (2)	Manna gum (1)
Scillae or scilliticae pilule (1)	Mercury (1)	Marini, spiritus salis (1)
Seneca or senega or seneka (2)	Mirabile, sal (2)	Medicine, not specified (1)
Senna (1)	Myrrh (2)	Mochlica, unspecified (2)
Serpentaria (1)	Niter, unknown (1)	Muriaticus, sal (1)
Stomachic, not specified (1)	Oliva, oil (1)	Niter, spirit of (2)
Succinum, salt (2)	Ophthamia, aqua (2)	Niter, unknown (1)
Surgery, no meds (1)	Opium (1)	Nitrosi, spiritus aetheris (3)
Tartar emetic (4)	Opodeldoc or Steer's (3)	Oliva, oil (1)
Tartar solution (2)	Panacea, not specified (5)	Ophthalmia, aqua (3)
Thebaica, tinctura (1)	Peru, balsam (1)	Oxymel, scilli (1)
Trebintha, oil (1)	Pyrethrum (1)	Pectoral mixture/powder/balsam (1)
Unguent, unknown (3)	Ricini, oil (2)	Plaster, unspecified or unknown (2)
Unguentum, basilicon (2)	Saturni, cerate (2)	Quassia or Excelsa (7)
Uguentum, lytharm? (1)	Scillae or scilliticae pilule (2)	Rhei (7)
Unknown (3)	Senna (3)	Sapo albus [hispanus] (1)
Vermifuge, unspecified (3)	Sermaceti (1)	Saturn, extract of or cerussa acetate (6)
Vipera (3)	Serpentaria (6)	Seneca or senega or seneka (2)

Table 1.11. Ingredients and procedures (*continued*)

SEPTEMBER 1786–FEBRUARY 1791 INGREDIENT (*times prescribed*)	JUNE 1804–MARCH 1806 INGREDIENT (*times prescribed*)	JUNE 1825–AUGUST 1828 INGREDIENT (*times prescribed*)
Vitriol, elixir (1)	Soda or barilli (1)	Senna (6)
Vitriol, oil (1)	Stomachic, not specified (1)	Soda or barilla (6)
Volatile salts (1)	Sulphur, flowers of (2)	Specific amara (1)
	Suppurativum, unguentum (1)	Spermaceti (2)
	Surgery (5)	Stomachic, not specified (7)
	Tartar emetic (2)	Sulphus cupri or blue vitriol (4)
	Terebintha, oil (2)	Surgery (1)
	Unguent, not specified (1)	Tartar emetic (6)
	Unguentum, basilicon (2)	
	Unguentum, lytharm? (1)	
	Uva ursi (1)	
	Valerian radix (1)	
	Vermifuge, unspecified (4)	
	Vessicativum, tincture (1)	
	Vitriol, elixir (1)	
	Vitriol blue or sulphas cupri (2)	
	Volatile, liniment (2)	
	Volatile, salts (2)	
	Winteranus (3)	

Table 3.1. Moses Mosman's account books, payments received, Sudbury, MA

TYPE OF PAYMENT	ENTRIES/TOTAL ENTRIES	PERCENTAGE OF TOTAL
Cash		
1763–1789[1]	393/1197	33
1802–1820	265/802	33
Goods, services, labor		
1763–1789	388/1197	32
1802–1820	96/802	12
Notes		
1763–1789	54/1197	5
1802–1820	112/802	14
"Received in full" or in part		
1763–1789	127/1197	11
1802–1820	310/802	39
Adjustments to account (vial or medicine returned, or error)		
1763–1789	220/1197	18
1802–1820	14/802	2
Sold or transferred to third party		
1763–1789	12/1197	1
1802–1820	2/802	<1
Patient paid doctor's debt via a third party		
1763–1789	2/1197	<1
1802–1820	3/802	<1

Source: Moses Mosman, Account books, 1763–1820, American Antiquarian Society, Worcester, MA.

Notes: Percentage totals may not reach 100 due to rounding.

1. I was unable to classify two entries in the 1763–1789 book due to confusing language.

Table 3.2. Edward Flint's account books, payments received, Worcester, MA

TYPE OF PAYMENT	ENTRIES/TOTAL ENTRIES	PERCENTAGE OF TOTAL
Cash		
1766–1790	692/1377	50
1795–1816	371/754	49
Goods, services, labor		
1766–1790	434/1377	32
1795–1816	123/754	16
Notes		
1766–1790	108/1377	8
1795–1816	120/754	16
"Received in full" or in part		
1766–1790	40/1377	3
1795–1816	59/754	8
Adjustments to account (vial or medicine returned, or error)		
1766–1790	62/1377	5
1795–1816	60/754	8
Sold or transferred to third party		
1766–1790	22/1377	2
1795–1816	17/754	2
Patient paid doctor's debt via a third party		
1766–1790	18/1377	1
1790–1816	3/754	<1

Source: Moses Mosman, Account books, 1763–1820, American Antiquarian Society, Worcester, MA.

Note: Percentage totals may not reach 100 due to rounding.

Table 3.3. William Williams's account books, payments received, Deerfield, MA

TYPE OF PAYMENT	ENTRIES/TOTAL ENTRIES	PERCENTAGE OF TOTAL
Cash		
1787–1828[1]	58/282	21
1807–1828	99/854	12
Goods, services, labor		
1787–1828	205/282	73
1807–1828	704/854	82
Notes		
1787–1828	6/282	2
1807–1828	20/854	2
"Received in Full" or in part		
1787–1828	3/282	1
1807–1828	2/854	<1
Adjustments to account (vial or medicine returned, or error)		
1787–1828	5/282	2
1807–1828	17/854	2
Sold or transferred to a third party		
1787–1828	4/282	1
1795–1816	4/854	<1
Patient paid doctor's debt via third party		
1787–1828	0/1377	0
1795–1816	0/754	0

Source: William Stoddard Williams, account books, vols. 1–2, PMVA.

Notes: Percentage totals may not reach 100 due to rounding.

1. The account books overlap in dates because patients listed in the 1787–1828 book continued to make payments up until 1828. Archivists often catalog using the first date noted and the last date listed. As with Mosman, I analyzed ninety pages. The 1807–1828 account book was three times the length of the 1787–1828 book, with the same small handwriting, thus I did only thirty pages of that book. In both books, the patients' accounts are not listed alphabetically but in the order they were treated. Subsequent treatments are listed on the same page until space no longer allowed; Williams then made note of on which page the account continued.

Table 3.4. Nonpayment by patients, John G. Metcalf, Mendon, MA

REASONS FOR NONPAYMENT	PATIENTS	PERCENTAGE OF 280 TOTAL PATIENTS[1]
Poverty	87	31
Left town, absconded, removed	83	30
Death	73	26
Refusal to pay	11	4
Went to war	10	4
"Being soft" or "gone to pot"	4	1
Outlawed	3	1
By [his] charity	3	1
Bankrupt	2	1
By endorsement	2	1
Town ordered	2	1

Source: John George Metcalf, Ledger, 1844–83, Francis C. Wood Institute of the History of Medicine, College of Physicians, Philadelphia, PA.

Notes: Total percentage exceeds 100 due to rounding.

1. Of the 475 patient accounts listed in the ledger, 280 had partial or full amounts written off. Many of the amounts written off were in the $1–3 range, the highest being $122.99.

Table 3.5. Occupational classification of patients admitted to the MGH

OCCUPATION	1820s % OF 231	1830s % OF 269	1840s % OF 266
Professionals (attorney, clergyman, physician)	5	3	2
Commercial proprietors (builder, merchant, grocer, storekeeper, hatter)	6	4	2
Commercial employees (agent, bookkeeper, clerk)	1	1	2
Public service (constable, teacher, soldier)	1	1	1
Agriculture (farmer, gardener)	3	5	4
Skilled trade (baker, blacksmith, butcher, dentist, nurse, carpenter, painter, tailor, shipwright)	17	17	12
Semiskilled and service jobs (domestic, porter, stage driver, mariner, servant)	21	42	39
General laborer	14	8	15
Women (married, single, widowed)[1]	13	12	14
Misc. (actor, public singer, student, peddler, miner)	1	5	7
Unknown (cotton garder, restaurateur, Brattleman, operative)	0	<1	<1
No occupation given	17	4	2

Source: Records of the Massachusetts General Hospital, 1824–1915, vols. 3, 13, 24, 34, 44, 54, 64, 74, 84, 94, 104, 114, 124, 134, 144, 154, 164, Francis C. Countway Library of Medicine, Boston, MA.

Notes: These classifications are based on those constructed by Michael B. Katz. I am not determining social mobility but how each patient identified his/her occupation and what that tells us about shifts in people who sought treatment in a hospital, for which a structural classification is more than adequate for my needs. For debates on occupational classifications, see Michael B. Katz, "Occupational Classification in History," *Journal of Interdisciplinary History* 3, no. 1 (Summer 1972): 63–88; Stuart Blumin, "The Historical Study of Vertical Mobility," *Historical Methods Newsletter* 1, no.1 (1968): 1–13; and Clyde Griffen, "Occupational Mobility in Nineteenth-Century America: Problems and Possibilities, *Journal of Social History* 5, no. 3 (Spring 1972): 310–30.

1. House physicians would designate female patients by their marital status. Other females who were designated as "single domestic" were counted under the occupational category of semiskilled/service.

Table 5.1. List of plaintiffs

NAME	OCCUPATION	SOURCE OF INFORMATION ON OCCUPATION
Ashworth, John	On behalf of son, picker in woolen mill	*Ashworth, Jr. v. Kittridge* (66 Mass. 193; 1853 Mass, Lexus 211; 12 CUSH 193)
Barber, Azel W.	Shoe finisher	Of Brookline, MA; 1868 Brookline City Directory
Blanche, Mrs. E.	Maker of wax flowers	1868 Pittsfield, MA City Directory
Conant, Francis	Farmer, value of real estate $3500	Of Stow, MA; 1850 U.S. Federal Census, age 61
Delaware, L. C.	Farmer	1892 Newburyport City Directory; Lyman C. Delaware, born 1823
Edgely, Emma	Unknown	
Harris, Louis	Cigar maker	"New England News Items," *Springfield Weekly Republican,* March 9, 1867, 8
Haskell, Elias	Master mariner	1873 Newburyport City Directory
Hayden, Benjamin F.	Worked in boot factory	Of Braintree, MA; 1870 U.S. Federal Census
Hennessey, John	Boat builder	1870 U.S. Federal Census for John P. Hennessey of Chelsea, MA
Hibbard, Emery	Blacksmith	1872 Lowell, MA, City Directory
Howard, Barzilla	Unknown	Of Portland?
Howe, Mrs.	Unknown	
Kerr, John	Unknown	Of Franklin, MA
Maynard, David	Baggage maker	1874 Clinton, MA, City Directory for David H. Maynard
McTeager	Domestic	"City and Vicinity," *Lowell Daily Citizen and News,* September 18, 1865, 2
Moody, Willard	Mason, value of real estate $1600	Of Williamstown, MA; 1850 U.S. Federal Census, age 56
Noyes, Moses L.	Peddler	"Case of Mal-practice," *BMSJ* 54, no. 6 (March 13, 1856), 109
Rice	Ship's carpenter	"Another Suite [sic] for Mal-practice," *BMSJ* 51, no. 25 (January 17, 1855), 504.
Rice, Abel	Unknown	Of Adams, MA
Reynolds, H. E.	Unknown	
Smith, Thomas D.	Unknown	
Stackpole	Unknown	Of Charlestown, MA
Tirell, G. W.	Unknown	Of Methuen, MA
Twombly	Wife of invalid husband	"Suburban items," *Boston Daily Atlas,* January 23, 1852, 1
Volmuth, Augustus	German gunsmith	"Trial for Malpractice," *BMSJ* 51, no. 6 (March 13, 1856), 109
Waite, John	Master harness maker	Of Palmer, MA; 1860 U.S. Federal Census, age 59
Wilson, Jane (5)	2 kept house; 1 domestic; 1 cotton mill; 1 no occupation listed	5 listed in Worcester County (Ancestry.com)

APPENDIX A

Self-Medication Data

The following are data for cases in which the house physician clearly indicates that the patient had not received prior medical advice for treating the illness that drove him/her to seek treatment at MGH. Statements that a patient was not receiving medical advice or was self-treating included "was in the habit of taking," "was not under medical treatment," "took medicine without medical advice," or "took medicine." Phrases that indicated a patient was under medical care included "called in a physician when he worsened," "account given by Dr.," "by direction of physician," or "was given medicine." In some instances, it was unclear whether the medicine a patient took had been prescribed by a physician. Often patients were not taking any medicine at all. In some cases, initially the patient was not under a doctor's care and self-medicated for the complaint, then sought physicians' advice before entering the hospital. I recorded medicines that were clearly indicated as self-medications and were specifically for the treatment of the symptoms that brought them to the MGH.

1820s

Number of patients who self-medicated in sampled records: 152
  No medication 64 (42%)
  Cathartics 43 (28%)[1]
  Medicine, not specified 17 (11%)
  Emetics 16 (11%)
  Wound care 8 (5%)
  Other, including anti-venereal 4, bleeding 1, and narcotics 5 (7%)
  SOURCE: Records of Massachusetts General Hospital (MGH), vols. 2, 3, 13, 24, and 34, Francis A. Countway Medical Library, Boston (hereafter Countway).

1830s

Number of patients who self-medicated in sample records: 199
  No medication 113 (57%)
  Cathartics 51 (26%)[2]
  Emetics 19 (10%)
  Wound care 19 (10%)
  Medicines, not specified 13 (7%)
  Other, including bleeding 6, usually local with leeches or cupping; and narcotics 5 (5%)
  Source: Records of MGH, vols. 44, 54, 64, 74, 84, and 94, Countway.

1840s

Number of patients who self-medicated in sampled records: 160
  No medicine 98 (61%)
  Cathartics 36 (23%)
  Medicines, not specified 23 (14%)
  Emetics 15 (9%)
  Wound care 14 (9%)
  Other, including narcotic 9, bleeding 1, and anti-venereal 1 (7%)
  Source: Records of MGH vols. 104, 114, 124, 134, 144, and 154, Countway.

Notes

1. Mostly, cathartics were unspecified (26) but many of a strong-acting type such as mercury or calomel were used (8). Of the mild variety, patients took aloes, myrrh, and saline mixtures.
2. Of the reports of cathartics taken by patients, most were "not specified" and salt water. Castor oil appears to have increased in popularity.

APPENDIX B

Diagnosis Tables for the 1820s, 1830s, and 1840s: Newly Admitted Patients at MGH

Tables list only patients for whom a diagnosis was recorded. They are recorded as they were written. In some volumes, the house physician included the "vulgar name" for the ailment. Some patients received several diagnoses, and each diagnosis has been recorded in its appropriate category using John Mason Good, *The Study of Medicine* (Boston: Wells & Lily, 1823); note that hysteria is categorized as a disease of the nervous functions because doctors understood it as a condition of overly excited nerves. Total percentage is 110% due to patients with more than one diagnosis.

Table A1. The 1820s
(total number of patients diagnosed with ailments in sampled volumes: 229)

DIAGNOSIS	PATIENTS RECORDED
Fever	
Anetus quotidianus (quotidian ague or intermittent fever)	5
Anetus tertianus (tertian ague)	1
Enecia cauma (inflammatory fever)	15
Enecia typhus or typhus	12
Fever, chills	10
Rheumatic fever	1
Synochus fever (continuous fever)	9
Total (percentage)	53 (23%)
Respiratory Disorders	
Affectation of the lung	1
Affliction of the lungs	1
Bex humida (wet cough)	2
Bronchitis	8
Chest pains/hemoptysis/cough blood	11
Cough	7
Dyspnoea (difficulty breathing)	1
Difficulty breathing	2
Empresma pneumonitis or pneumonia	6
Phthisis pulmonitis (consumption)	8
Respiratory or pulmonary complaint	2
Total (percentage)	49 (21%)

Table A1. The 1820s (*continued*)

DIAGNOSIS	PATIENTS RECORDED
Gastrointestinal Disorders	
Acid reflux	1
Cardialgia (heartburn)	1
Diarrhea	4
Disease of the stomach	1
Dyspepsia or limosis (indigestion)	12
Dysentery	2
Costive or constipation	4
Gastritis	1
Peritonitis (inflammation of)	2
Vomiting	2
Total (percentage)	30 (13%)
Joint Disease or Pain	
Acute rheumatism	2
Arthrosia, chronic (degenerative joints)	2
Arthritis	3
Arthrosia acuta	3
Rheumatism	12
Total (percentage)	22 (10%)
Diseases of the Nervous Functions	
Alusia (hallucinations)	1
Body numbness, acute	1
Cephalitis (inflammation of the brain)	1
Epilepsy	5
Hemiplegia	1
Palsy	2
Paralysis	9
Total (percentage)	20 (9%)
General Pain: Skeletal, Bodily, or Headaches	
Back pain, injury	1
Body pain, acute	3
Body pain, general	5
Cephalea or intense headache	7
Injury	1
Pleuralgia, chronic (chronic pain in chest)	2
Total (percentage)	19 (8%)
Skin Diseases	
Cutaneous affection	1
Impetigo	2
Lapidosis psoriasis or psoriasis	5
Swelling and rash	2
Total (percentage)	10 (4%)

Table A1. The 1820s (*continued*)

DIAGNOSIS	PATIENTS RECORDED
Venereal Diseases	
Genital sore	1
Syphilis	7
Syphilis, secondary	1
Total (percentage)	9 (4%)
Female Disorders	
Amenorrhea (absence of menses)	2
Chronic menses	1
Dysmenorrhea (painful menses)	2
Paramenia (irregular menses)	1
Vaginal discharge	1
Total (percentage)	8 (3%)
Behavioral or Mental Disorders	
Delirium	1
Disorder of animal functions	1
Ebrious (excessive drinking)	1
Euphoria melancholia (excitable, depressive)	1
Hypochondria	2
Mania	1
Total (percentage)	7 (3%)
Cardiovascular Disorders	
Chest pain	1
Chronic palpitations	2
Hypertrophy of heart	1
Total (percentage)	4 (2%)
Other	
Anasarca (general swelling of the skin)	1
Anemia	1
Colic	3
Debilitated	1
Dropsy, not specified	1
Empresmus otitis (ear inflammation)	2
Eye or ophthalmia	1
Hepatitis, acute and chronic	4
Jaundice	2
Maramus (malnutrition)	1
Scrofula (swelling of lymph nodes in neck)	1
Total (percentage)	20 (9%)
Cancers	
Tumor	3
Total (percentage)	3 (1%)

Table A1. The 1820s (*continued*)

DIAGNOSIS	PATIENTS RECORDED
Urinary Disorders	
Painful urination	1
Cystitis, inflammation of the bladder	1
Total (percentage)	2 (<1%)
Unknown	
Mimosa chronica	1
Syspasia hypertension (spasms of the vessels?)	1
Total (percentage)	2 (<1%)

Table A2. The 1830s
(total number of patients diagnosed with ailments in sampled volumes: 269)

DIAGNOSIS	PATIENTS RECORDED
Fever	
Anetus quotidianus (quotidian ague/intermittent fever)	6
Enecia cauma (inflammatory fever)	3
Enecia typhus	43
Intermittent fever	1
Scarlet fever	1
Synochus fever (continuous fever)	9
Typhoid fever	1
Total (percentage)	64 (24%)
Respiratory Disorders	
Asthma	2
Bex humida (wet cough)	3
Bex sicca (dry cough)	1
Bronchitis	7
Chest pains/hemoptysis/coughing blood	1
Cough	3
Disease of lung	1
Dropsy of chest	1
Dyspnoea (difficulty breathing)	2
Empresma pneumonitis or pneumonia	10
Gangrene of lung	1
Marasmus pulmonitis or phthisis (consumption)	10
Pleurisy	5
Pulmonary tubercles	1
Total (percentage)	48 (18%)

Table A2. The 1830s (*continued*)

DIAGNOSIS	PATIENTS RECORDED
Gastrointestinal Disorders	
Cholera	1
Costive or constipation	2
Diarrhea	4
Dyspepsia or limosis (indigestion)	20
Dysentery or diarrhea chronic	5
Gastritis	1
Hydrops abdomen (dropsy of abdominal cavity)	1
Neuralgia abdominalis	1
Polyposa, aedoptosis (?)	1
Ulera vitiosa (ulcers)	1
Total (percentage)	37 (14%)
Joint Disease or Pain	
Arthrosia, chronic, or chronic rheumatism	9
Arthritis	1
Arthrosia acuta, or acute rheumatism	13
Rheumatism	3
Total (percentage)	26 (10%)
Female Disorders	
Amenorrhea (absence of menses)	2
Dysmenorrhea (painful menses)	2
Menorrhagia acuta (uterine hemorrhage)	4
Neuralgia uteri (irritable womb)	1
Oedoptosis uteri (falling of womb)	1
Paramenia (irregular menses)	4
Prolapsed uterus	1
H. Uterine (?)	1
"Whites" or leucorrhea (vaginal discharge)	2
Total (percentage)	18 (7%)
Diseases of the Nervous Functions	
Disease of the brain	2
Hysteria	4
Epilepsy	2
Palsy	7
Sinus vertigo (dizziness)	1
Total (percentage)	16 (6%)
General Pain: Skeletal, Bodily, or Headaches	
Cephalea or intense headache	7
Cephalea gravans (stupid headache)	1
Cachexies or dysthetica (burning pain)	1
Hemicranias (migraine)	1
Neuralgia pedi	1
Total (percentage)	11 (4%)

Table A2. The 1830s (*continued*)

DIAGNOSIS	PATIENTS RECORDED
Skin Diseases	
Disease of skin	1
Ecthyma	1
Eczema	2
Exanthesis urticaria	1
Hemorrhoids	1
Impetigo	1
Lapidosis psoriasis or psoriasis	1
Repelled eruption	1
Total (percentage)	10 (4%)
Behavioral or Mental Disorders	
Alusia hypochondria	6
Delirium tremens (insanity)	3
Total (percentage)	9 (3%)
Cardiovascular Disorders	
Chronic palpitations	2
Empresma peritonitis (inflammation of peritoneum)	1
Morbus cordis (heart disease)	2
Phlebitis (inflamed vein)	1
Total (percentage)	6 (2%)
Venereal Diseases	
Gonorrhea	1
Syphilis	3
Total (percentage)	4 (1%)
Urinary Disorders	
Painful urination	1
Paruria melita (diabetes or saccharine urine)	1
Total (percentage)	2 (<1%)
Cancers	
Tumor	1
Total (percentage)	1 (<1%)

Table A2. The 1830s (continued)

DIAGNOSIS	PATIENTS RECORDED
Other	
Anasarca (general swelling of skin)	1
Catarrhus communis (cold in the head)	2
Chlorosis (green sickness)	1
Colic	1
Chorea (involuntary movements)	1
Dysphonia susurraus (loss of voice)	1
Elephantiasis (leg)	1
Empresmus otitis (ear inflammation)	1
Hepatitis, acute and chronic	1
Inflammation of leg	1
Marasmus (malnutrition)	1
Periostitis sterni (inflammation of sternum)	1
Purpura hem. (land scurvy)	1
Total (percentage)	14 (5%)

Table A3. The 1840s
(total number of patients diagnosed with ailments in sampled volumes: 265)

DIAGNOSIS	PATIENTS RECORDED
Respiratory Disorders	
Bronchitis	8
Cough	1
Empresma pneumonitis or pneumonia	9
Emphysema	2
Gangrene of lungs	2
Haemoptysis (coughing blood)	1
Marasmus phthisis (consumption)	29
Pleurisy	5
Pulmonary disease	1
Tubules of the lungs	3
Total (percentage)	61 (23%)
Fever	
Bilious remittent fever	1
Fever, chills	7
Intermittent fever	6
Lynochus (summer fever)	1
Synochus fever	1
Typhoid fever	23
Total (percentage)	39 (15%)

Table A3. The 1840s (*continued*)

DIAGNOSIS	PATIENTS RECORDED
Gastrointestinal Disorders	
Ascites (fluid in abdominal cavity or the coelum)	2
Chronic diarrhea	10
Derangement of the stomach	2
Dyspepsia or limosis (indigestion)	11
Dysentery	10
Gastritis	1
Hematemesis (vomiting blood)	1
Intestinal irritation	1
Stomach disorder	1
Total (percentage)	39 (15%)
Diseases of the Nervous Functions	
Cerebral disease or disease of the brain	7
Chorea (tremors, St. Vitus's dance)	2
Epilepsy	2
Hemiplegia	3
Hysteria	1
Meningitis, acute	1
Neuralgia (nerve ache)	5
Paralysis	6
Paraplegia	5
Sciatica	2
Tubercular meningitis	2
Total (percentage)	36 (14%)
Joint Disease or Pain	
Acute rheumatism	6
Chronic rheumatism	14
Disease of the knee joint	1
Rheumatism	1
Total (percentage)	22 (8%)
Other	
Affection of liver or cirrhosis	3
Cachexia (malnutrition)	1
Cynanche (severe sore throat)	1
Debilitation	1
Dropsy, not specified	2
Elephantiasis	1
Jaundice (obstruction of liver)	3
Laryngitis	1
Loss of consciousness	1
Otorrhea (discharge from ear)	1
Periostatis sterni (inflammation of sternum)	1
Scrofula (swelling of lymph nodes in neck)	1
Sycosis (tubercles of face)	1
Tubera of liver	1
Total (percentage)	19 (7%)

Table A3. The 1840s (*continued*)

DIAGNOSIS	PATIENTS RECORDED
Female Disorders	
Amenorrhea (absence of menses)	4
Chlorosis (anemia due to menses, "green sickness")	2
Disease of uterine	1
Irritable uterus	1
Menorrhagia active (uterine hemorrhage)	1
Paramenia (irregular menses)	1
Prolapsed uterus	1
Total (percentage)	11 (4%)
General Pain: Skeletal, Bodily, or Headaches	
Back pain, injury	1
Body pain, general	1
Disease of the bones	1
Disease of the spine	1
Intense headaches	3
Total (percentage)	7 (3%)
Skin Diseases	
Cutaneous disease	1
Eczema	3
Erysipelas (skin infection)	1
Lichen (type of rash)	1
Psoriasis	1
Scabies	1
Tinea capitis (ringworm of the scalp)	1
Total (percentage)	9 (3%)
Behavioral or Mental Disorders	
Ebrious (excessive drinking)	1
Hypochondria	2
Mania	1
Total (percentage)	4 (2%)
Cardiovascular Disorders	
Disease of the heart	4
Phlebitis (inflammation of the vein)	1
Total (percentage)	5 (2%)
Cancers	
Abdominal tumor	3
Cancer of the stomach	1
Carcinoma, not specified	1
Carcinoma of the liver	1
Total (percentage)	6 (2%)
Urinary Diseases	
Diabetes	1
Disease of kidneys	2
Dysuria (painful urination)	3
Hematuria (blood in urine)	1
Total (percentage)	7 (3%)

Table A3. The 1840s (*continued*)

DIAGNOSIS	PATIENTS RECORDED
Venereal diseases	
Secondary syphilis	3
Total (percentage)	3 (1%)
Unknown	
Effects of cold water	1
Total (percentage)	1 (<1%)

APPENDIX C

List of Massachusetts Cases Identified

1828 *Rice v. Bassett;* regarding care of wound on knee; verdict for defendant; "Law and Surgery," *Massachusetts Spy,* October 10, 1833, 2.

1847 *Howard v. Grover;* regarding amputation; verdict for plaintiff; "Damages for Mal-Practice," *Massachusetts Spy,* December 15, 1847, 3.

1847 *Delaware v. Gale;* regarding criminal prosecution of malpractice in delivery; verdict for defendant and case dismissed; "Trial of Physician for Assault and Battery," *Boston Medical and Surgical Journal* (hereafter *BMSJ*) 38, no. 26 (July 26, 1848), 528. Case tried in New Hampshire, as that was where the plaintiff's lived. Physician was from Salisbury Mills, Massachusetts.

1847 Unnamed Parties; regarding deformed finger; verdict for defendant; "Law and Surgery," *Salem Registrar,* May 24, 1847, 2.

1849 *Conant v. Manning;* regarding dislocation; verdict for plaintiff; "Prosecution for Mal-Practice," *BMSJ* 40, no. 16 (May 23, 1849), 318, and "Trial for Mal-P," *BMSJ* 42, no. 5 (February 27, 1850), 79.

1851 *Smith v. Hyndeman and Fowle;* regarding not specified; verdict unknown; "Supreme Judicial Court," *Boston Evening Transcript,* September 30, 1851, 2.

1852 *Moody v. Sabin;* regarding fracture; verdict for defendant; appealed, exceptions overruled; 63 Mass. 505 (1852).

1853 *Twombly v. Leach,* and 65 Mass. 397 LEXIS 118 (1853); regarding amputation of thumb; verdict for plaintiff; appealed, granted new trial; "Prosecution for Mal-Practice," *BMSJ* 45, no. 10 (October 8, 1851), 203; "News," *Boston Evening Transcript,* January 22, 1852, 2; "Suburban Items," *Boston Daily Atlas,* January 23, 1852, 1.

1853 *Ashworth v. Kittridge* [no number in orginal], 66 Mass. 193 LEXIS 211 (October 1853), regarding wound care, verdict for plaintiff; court set aside; "Prosecution for Mal-Practice," *BMSJ* 48, no. 14 (May 4, 1853), 281; "Mal-practice Case—Verdict Set Aside," *Salem Registrar,* May 8, 1854, 2; "Things in General," *Boston Courier,*

December 18, 1854, 4; and "Dr. Kittredege, Newburyport, Rendered," *Salem Registrar,* December 18, 1854, 2.

1854   *Edgely v. Bartlett;* regarding bone setting; verdicts for three trials in which two juries did not reach agreement and third jury found for defendant; "Prosecution for Mal-Practice," *BMSJ* 51, no. 5 (November 8, 1854), 305, and "News and Miscellaneous Items," *Boston Evening Transcript,* November 9, 1854, 1.

1854   *Kerr v. Perry;* regarding dislocated shoulder; verdict for defendant; "Things in General," *Boston Courier,* February 27, 1854, 2.

1855   *Rice v. Thorndike;* regarding amputation; verdict for plaintiff; "Another Suit of Mal-Practice,"*BMSJ* 51, no. 25 (January 17, 1855), 504.

1856   *Volmuth v. Hathaway;* regarding fracture; verdict for defendant; "Trial for Mal-Practice," *BMSJ* 56, no. 1 (February 5, 1857), 101, and "Items," *Massachusetts Spy,* February 25, 1857, 3.

1856   *Noyes v. Allen;* regarding fracture; verdict for defendant; "Case of Mal-Practice Tried," *BMSJ* 54, no. 6 (March 13 1856), 109, and "News and Miscellaneous Items," *Boston Evening Transcript,* January 21, 1856, 1.

1859   *Tirell v. Haynes;* regarding setting of arm; verdicts: two trials with undecided jury; "Suit for Mal-Practice," *Lowell Daily Citizen and News,* May 28, 1859, 2.

1860   *Waite v. Higgins;* regarding crippled boy; verdict unknown; "General News," *Massachusetts Spy,* May 9, 1860, 3.

1860   *Reynolds v. Gile;* regarding injuries not specified; case dismissed for insufficient evidence; "Superior Court," *Salem Registrar,* June 18, 1860, 2.

1865   *Barber v. Merriam,* 93 Mass. 322 LEXIS 263 (1865).; regarding an illness; verdict for plaintiff; appealed, exceptions overruled.

1865   *Blanche v. Cole;* regarding setting of shoulder; verdict for plaintiff; "New England News Items," *Springfield Weekly Republican,* June 10, 1865, 8; "Mrs. E. Blanche," *Pittsfield Sun,* June 15, 1865, 2; and "Damages for Mal-Practice," *Boston Daily Journal,* March 9, 1866, 2.

1865   *McTeager v. Brown;* regarding broken limbs; verdict unknown; "City and Vicinity," *Lowell Daily Citizen and News,* September 18, 1865, 2.

1867   *Harris v. Comins;* regarding treatment of "stricture" (possibly urethal); verdict unknown; "New England News Items," *Springfield Weekly Republican,* March 9, 1867, 8.

1867   *Howe v. Barnes;* regarding a broken arm; verdict for plaintiff; "From Our Second Evening Edition from Yesterday," *Boston Daily Journal,* May 7, 1867, 2.

1869   Unnamed Parties; regarding a broken limb; verdict for defendant; "Suits for Mal-Practice," *Boston Daily Journal,* May 22, 1869, 2.

1870   *Maynard v. Symonds and Burdett;* regarding an amputated wrong finger; verdict unknown; "Suit for Malpractice," *Boston Daily Journal,* April 30, 1869, 2.

1870   *Wilson v. Symonds;* regarding a broken finger, splintered wrong finger, both fingers deformed; verdict for plaintiff; "Curious Case," *Lowell Citizen and News,* April 30, 1870, 2.

1871   *Hennessey v. Wheeler and Bean;* regarding the amputation of wrong finger; verdict for plaintiff; "Verdict in Medical Malpractice Case," *Lowell Daily Citizen and News,* February 4, 1871, 1.

1872   *Hibbard v. Thompson,* 109 Mass. 286 LEXIS 55 (1872); regarding treatment of rheumatism; verdict for defendant; appealed exceptions overruled.

1872   *Unnamed plaintiff v. Millard of North Adams;* regarding fracture of thigh; verdict unknown; "North Adams," *Pittsfield Sun,* October 30, 1872, 3.

1873   *Hayden v. Babbitt;* regarding injuries not specified; verdict jury undecided; "Dedham an Alleged Case of Malpractice," *Boston Evening Journal,* January 25, 1873, 4.

1873   *Stackpole v. Fuller;* regarding a broken wrist; verdict unknown; "City and Vicinity," *Lowell Daily Citizen and News,* March 24, 1873, 2.

1873   *Haskell et ux v. Enoch Cross;* regarding setting of son's broken arm; verdict for plaintiff; "Supreme Judicial Court," *Salem Register,* April 28, 1873, 2.

APPENDIX D

Criminal Cases in Massachusetts

1849   Dr. John Stevens of Boston, found not guilty of manslaughter by a jury in the death of Ann Gallagher, "Dr. John Stevens—Municipal," *Gloucester Telegraph,* March 28, 1849, 2.

1851   Dr. T. P. Smith, tried for manslaughter of two children by malpractice, "The Manslaughter Trial," *Boston Evening Transcript,* April 23, 1851, 3.

1855   Mrs. Goodwin, midwife, arrested and tried for the death of Mrs. Samuel Breckenridge. After delivery of a child, mistook an inverted uterus for a tumor and cut it out; the patient bled to death before doctor arrived. "Malpractice," *Barre Patriot,* August 24, 1855, 2.

1860   *Commonwealth v. Tilton;* jury of inquest in Haverhill returned verdict against Dr. James A. Tilton of Newburyport for the death of Caroline Roswell during an unlawful operation; "The Case of Malpractice at Haverhill," *Boston Courier,* May 24, 1860, 1.

1867   William H. White; Springfield, Mass; arrested in the death of Elizabeth Metbren after performing an abortion; "Arrest for Malpractice—A Swindler," *Boston Daily Journal,* August 14, 1867, 4.

1868   Dr. Charles P. Powers, charged with causing the death of Mrs. Mary A. Bowen on August 5, "Boston and Vicinity," *Lowell Daily Citizen and News,* August 22, 1868, 2.

1870   Dr. Samuel F. Batchelder, indicted for manslaughter for the death of Martha E. Hall; "Boston and Vicinity Runaway Accidents," *Boston Daily Journal,* February 15, 1870, 2.

1872   Charles H. Scholes, posing as a physician, charged with the death of Sarah E. Brown in suspected abortion, "Death from Malpractice," *Lowell Daily Citizen and News,* May 29, 1872, 2.

1872   Dr. Hill of Boston, charged in the death of a domestic by the name of O'Brien, "New England News Summary," *Massachusetts Spy,* December 13, 1872, 4.

APPENDIX E

Methodologies Used

Methodology for Physicians' Account Books in Chapter 3

I reviewed all the payment entries for the credit side of the account book. For tables 3.1, 3.2, and 3.3, each mixed entry—those with goods, labor, and/or cash specified—I counted one entry of goods and labor and one entry for cash. In figure 1 (in chapter 3) I computed a value chart in order to analyze goods as a percentage of the total value collected. In both methods, payments in goods and labor decreased.

Methodology of Sampling for MGH Records

I recorded data for each newly admitted patient, which included his or her long health and personal history. I sampled every tenth volume, which covered the dates as indicated below:

1820s (236 total newly admitted patients sampled)
Vol. 3: February to August 1823; 41 new patients
Vol. 13: October to December 1825; 63 new patients
Vol. 24: July to September 1827; 54 new patients
Vol. 34: August to October 1829; 78 new patients

1830s (274 patients)
Vol. 44: August to October 1831; 59 new patients
Vol. 54: June to September 1833; 85 new patients
Vol. 64: March to April 1835; 35 new patients
Vol. 74: August to October 1836; 49 new patients
Vol. 84: November to December 1837; 23 new patients
Vol. 94: February to April 1839; 23 patients

1840s (271 patients)
Vol. 104: October 1840 to January 1841; 39 patients
Vol. 114: December 1842 to February 1843; 42 patients
Vol. 124: February to April 1845; 29 patients
Vol. 134: February to April 1847; 32 patients
Vol. 144: May to August 1848; 71 patients
Vol. 154: June to August 1849; 58 patients

NOTES

INTRODUCTION

1. William G. Rothstein, *American Physicians in the Nineteenth Century: From Sects to Science* (Baltimore: Johns Hopkins University Press, 1972), 50.
2. Galen posited that sickness occurred when the humors of the body (yellow bile, blood, phlegm, and black bile) were out of balance. For a brief, cogent summary of therapeutics, see Thomas A. Horrocks, *Popular Print and Popular Medicine: Almanacs and Health Advice in Early America* (Amherst: University of Massachusetts Press, 2009), 43–66.
3. From Boerhaave he adopted the concept that the body mimicked a machine, and broken machines cannot fix themselves. Yet Rush did not agree with Boerhaave's assessment that the root of illness derived from problems in the nervous system; he believed in Cullen's theory, which located the problem in the circulatory system. Within the circulatory system, Cullen argued for an iatrophysical view, in which spasms of the arteries produced "constriction" symptoms such as thirst and dry skin. A fever signaled that a state of debility had occurred. Brown took the concept of debility not as a symptom but as a diseased state that emerged as two types: direct debility (when stimuli such as heat, contagions, or emotions were too weak to balance the reaction of the body to the stimuli, or its "excitability") and indirect debility (when the stimuli were too strong and exhausted the body). Thus, direct debilities were treated with stimulants to attain balance. In cases of indirect debilities, depletive treatments, cold, and opiates were used to lessen the stimuli in order to achieve homeostasis. Rush decided that debility represented neither a symptom of disease nor a disease in itself, but was the cause of disease. In essence, Rush had simplified Brown's theory by proposing one state (which most mirrored Brown's indirect debility) as a cause of illness and treated it with a depletive system. Richard Shryock, *Medicine and Society in America, 1660–1860* (Ithaca, NY: Cornell University Press, 1960), 69. Rush believed that part of perfecting republican independence meant promoting original thinking. Forming "a complete system of [American] medicine" fit into achieving this goal; Paul E. Kopperman, "'Venerate

the Lancet': Benjamin Rush's Yellow Fever Therapy in Context," *Bulletin of the History of Medicine* 78 (Fall 2004): 571–73.
4. These ideas were based on Francis Bacon's inductive reasoning. John Harley Warner, *Against the Spirit of System: The French Impulse in Nineteenth-Century American Medicine* (Princeton: Princeton University Press, 1998), 165.
5. Warner, *Against the Spirit*, 246.
6. Paul Starr, *The Social Transformation of American Medicine* (New York: Basic Books, 1982); Martin S. Pernick, *A Calculus of Suffering: Pain, Professionalism, and Anesthesia in Nineteenth-Century America* (New York: Columbia University Press, 1985); Rothstein, *American Physicians;* and Shryock, *Medicine and Society.*
7. Mostly recently, Elaine G. Breslaw has depicted early American therapeutics as brutal and ineffective as they were practiced by a medical profession that was "unable to organize" and was "retarded by a vast army of illiterate and incompetent medical personnel." Elaine G. Breslaw, *Lotions, Potions, Pills, and Magic: Health Care in Early America* (New York: New York University Press, 2012), 185.
8. One study exists that focuses on one town: J. Worth Estes and David M. Goodman, *Changing Humors of Portsmouth: The Medical Biography of an American Town, 1623–1983* (Boston: F. A. Countway Library of Medicine, 1986); and several studies give evidence from all over, obscuring regional differences, such as Rothstein, *American Physicians in the Nineteenth Century.*
9. Alternative practitioners comprised a small percentage of health-care providers. Joseph Kett found that homeopathic and botanic physicians accounted for only one in ten physicians. Joseph Kett, *The Formation of the American Medical Profession: The Role of Institutions, 1780–1860* (New Haven: Yale University Press, 1968), 186. I will use the term "regular" interchangeably with "orthodox" and the term "irregular" with "unorthodox."
10. John Harley Warner, *The Therapeutic Perspective: Medical Practice, Knowledge, and Identity in America, 1820–1885* (Princeton: Princeton University Press, 1997), 2n.
11. Kenneth Allen DeVille, *Medical Malpractice in Nineteenth-Century America: Origins and Legacy* (New York: New York University Press, 1990), xii.

1. MEDICAL PRACTICE IN MASSACHUSETTS

1. Francis C. Woodworth, *A Peep at Our Neighbors* (New York: Charles Scribner, 1852), 50, 54.
2. Oliver Wendell Holmes, *Currents and Counter-Currents in Medical Science with Other Addresses and Essays* (Boston: Ticknor & Fields, 1861), 25–27.
3. Rush believed that part of perfecting the republican independence involved promoting original thinking. Forming "a complete system of [American] medicine" fit into achieving this goal; Paul E. Kopperman, "'Venerate the Lancet': Benjamin Rush's Yellow Fever Therapy in Context," *Bulletin of the History of Medicine* 78 (Fall 2004): 571–73.
4. Samuel Thomson, an itinerant physician, developed a system of medical practice

using botanic remedies outlined in his book, *New Guide to Health* (1822). Like Rush, Thomson believed that disease had one cause. In Thomson's mind that cause was loss of body heat. Removing the obstructed perspiration would restore it. Along with steaming, stimulant roots and herbs (especially lobelia) were employed to cleanse and invigorate the body through purging, vomiting, and perspiring. Part of what distinguished Thomson's botanic system from the therapeutics practiced by "regulars" was the lack of bleeding or use of mercurial drugs. His system differed from those of other rural botanical doctors because he provided a system of care that was comprised of an explanation of disease and a small, precisely ordered pharmacopoeia of herbal remedies. For more information on Thomsonian medicine, see Norman Gevitz, ed., *Other Healers: Unorthodox Medicine in America* (Baltimore: Johns Hopkins University Press, 1988).

Homeopathic medicine arose from the work of German physician and theorist, Samuel Christian Hahnemann. The therapeutic approach argued that a drug prescribed should be similar in action to the disease. This would produce in the body a secondary form of the same illness, but one the body could combat. Thus, the secondary form would assist the "vital powers" of the body to overcome the primary disease. Later, a second theory of infinitesimals was added, which stipulated that the smaller the dose of the drug prescribed, the more effective it would be in stimulating the vital powers. Martin Kaufman, *Homeopathy in America: The Rise and Fall of Medical Heresy* (Baltimore: Johns Hopkins University Press, 1971), 26. Expectant medical practitioners approached therapy cautiously, first allowing nature to heal. Ideally, empiricists prescribed gentle medicines to aid nature, not to aggressively intervene.

5. John Harley Warner, *The Therapeutic Perspective: The Medical Practice, Knowledge and Identity in America, 1820–1885* (Princeton: Princeton University Press, 1997), 32. Also see Warner's charts in chapter 4, "Therapeutic Change," for statistical comparisons of the Massachusetts General Hospital (MGH) and Commercial Hospital in Cincinnati (CHC).

6. Robert B. Sullivan, "Sanguine Practices: A Historical and Historiographic Reconsideration of Heroic Therapy in the Age of Rush," *Bulletin of the History of Medicine* 68 (Summer 1994): 233.

7. Mary Gardiner Lowell, September 1843, personal journal 1843–49, vol. 81, Francis Cabot Lowell II Papers, Massachusetts Historical Society, Boston (hereafter MHS).

8. Evidence exists that doctors in Philadelphia practiced expectant medicine as well. One physician advised James Stuart to spend seven to ten days at "the great pine swamp" because the change in environment would be good for his health. Likewise, Stuart's grandfather's doctor said that he "ought to have the mountain or sea air for a little time." James H. Stuart to Margaret S. Forster, August 22, 1846, Forster Family Papers, Francis Wood Institute, Philadelphia (hereafter Wood). By the 1840s, heroics fell out of favor in many regions, although Warner's study of the use of heroic depletive medicines such as calomel in CHC increased from the 1840s to the 1850s. A willingness to rely solely on alterations of environment and diet to aid

nature constitutes expectant therapeutics, but the use of alterations in environment and diet were not unique to the nineteenth century. Before the popularity of heroic therapeutics many eighteenth-century health guides or longevity texts suggested changes in "air, food and drink, motion and rest, sleep and wakefulness" as ways to preserve health. Lamar Riley Murphy, *Enter the Physician: The Transformation of Domestic Medicine, 1760–1860* (Tuscaloosa: University of Alabama Press, 1991), 9.

9. Joseph Sargent, medical records, 1840–41, American Antiquarian Society, Worcester, MA (hereafter AAS).

10. Account books refer to ledgers where physicians documented patient visits, treatments, and charges under account names. Daybooks refer to records of patient name, visits, treatments, and charges by date. Some account books and daybooks do not include treatments provided. For convenience's sake, I use the terms interchangeably.

11. William G. Rothstein, *American Physicians in the Nineteenth Century: From Sects to Science* (Baltimore: Johns Hopkins University Press, 1972), 45.

12. For example, if the computer-generated numbers list showed the number seven, I began at the first page of the account book and counted seven entries down. I recorded the random number, the page number of the account book, the patient's name, drugs prescribed, and any comments noted by physician into my database. See appendix E for a complete discussion.

13. Warner, *Therapeutic Perspective*, 140. Rothstein, *American Physicians*, 45.

14. Archivists date documents based on the first and last dates entered. Thus, Mosman's last account book had entries dated 1820 due to payment on patients' accounts made after his death.

15. By "conservatively," I mean that the physician was not likely to dose aggressively with strong compounds.

16. "The Late Dr. Lowe, of Ashburnham," *Boston Medical and Surgical Journal* 11, no. 19 (December 17, 1834): 306.

17. More biographical information on Williams is available on the Pocumtuck Valley Memorial Association Web site, www.memorialhall.mass.edu.

18. I chose one account book from before the 1790s (when Rush's influence on therapeutics began), one account book from the 1800s (when heroic therapeutics has been considered at its height of use), and his last account book covering the 1820s (when use of heroic therapeutics was under public attack).

19. He practiced from 1813 to 1853.

20. "Biographical Memoirs of Rev. John Williams," Pocumtuck Valley Memorial Association, www.memorialhall.mass.edu/collections.

21. Appleton's Cyclopaedia of American Biography, vol. 5 (New York: D. Appleton, 1888), 602.

22. Bloodletting refers to venesection (the opening of veins with a lancet, usually in the arm); wet cupping (placing a cup, from which the air had been evacuated by heat, over the treatment area); scarification (12 to 20 small cuts made in the skin over an area of about 1.5 to 2 square inches); and the use of leeches. J. Worth

Estes, *Dictionary of Protopharmacology: Therapeutic Practices, 1700–1850* (Canton, MA: Science History Publications, 1990), 28; and Audrey Davis and Toby Appel, *Bloodletting Instruments in the National Museum of History and Technology: Smithsonian Studies in History and Technology* 41 (Washington, DC: Smithsonian Institution Press, 1979).

23. Warner, *Therapeutic Perspective*, 30.
24. The findings found in this study on private practice correlate with those of J. Worth Estes. Estes studied four physicians' private practices—two from New Hampshire and two from Boston. The Boston physicians, William Aspinwall and David Townsend, showed low percentages of bleeding during the late eighteenth century (0.8% from 1782 to 1795 and 0% in 1784 to 1791, respectively). Estes' methodology differed from mine. He did a 10% sampling (every tenth microfilm frame or double page) for all but Townsend (30%), but it was not random. In other words, taking every tenth page may have produced an unintended bias, depending on whether the physician recorded treatments dispensed that day or under a patient's name. J. Worth Estes, "Therapeutic Practice in Colonial New England," in *Medicine in Colonial Massachusetts, 1620–1820,* ed. Philip Cash et al., vol. 57 (Boston: The Colonial Society of Massachusetts, 1980), 291, 303.
25. Another explanation for Massachusetts physicians using bleeding less frequently than those in Philadelphia for example, could be that the incidences of fever and inflammation were fewer in Massachusetts. Although Boston has been described as "probably the healthiest of large American cities," life expectancies there "were still five or six years lower than those in rural Massachusetts." If bleeding was used in cases of fever as heroic practitioners advocated, then I would have expected to see bleeding performed more often in Boston (where fevers spread faster due to crowded living conditions) than in rural Massachusetts. In this study, Snow in Boston bled 0.7 percent compared to William Williams in Deerfield at 4 percent, who was practicing during the same period. According to this comparison, the higher incidences of fever in the city did not correlate to higher numbers of treatment by bleeding. Also, there is no reason to believe that people in Massachusetts suffered less from conditions such as rheumatism than those in other regions of the country. Thus, low incidences of bleeding appear to be dependent on choices made by physicians and patients, not on lower occurrence of conditions for which bleeding was the preferred treatment among heroic practitioners. Jack Larkin, *The Reshaping of Everyday Life, 1790–1840* (New York: Harper & Row, 1988), 81.
26. James Parkinson, *Medical Admonitions to Families, Respecting the Preservation of Health and the Treatment of the Sick* (Portsmouth, NH: N. W. & W. Pierce, 1803), 81–82.
27. Sheila M. Rothman, *Living in the Shadow of Death: Tuberculosis and the Social Experience of Illness in American History* (New York: Basic Books, 1994), 109.
28. Joseph Sargent, June 30, 1840, medical records, 1840–41, AAS. See entry for Mr. Knowles on September 4, 1841, for another example.
29. Jane A. Winchester, M.D., "Introducing Stephen West Williams, M.D., First

President of the Franklin District Medical Society" (paper presented commemorating the 150th anniversary of the Franklin District Medical Society, April 25, 2001), Pocumtuck Valley Memorial Library, Deerfield, MA (hereafter PVMA).

30. Robert B. Sullivan argues that Rush's use of heavy bleeding during the 1793 yellow fever epidemic was influenced by his reading of John Mitchell's manuscript "describing his regimen during the yellow fever outbreak of 1741 in Virginia." In the early decades of the nineteenth century, bleeding became a treatment for several types of fevers, inflammatory diseases such as rheumatism, and local swelling due to injury. Sullivan, "Sanguine Practices," 217–18.

31. *Barn-yard Rhymes; showing what opinions The Turkey, The Cock, The Goose, and The Duck entertain of Allopathia, Homopathia* [sic]*, Electro-galvanism, and the Animalcule Doctrines* (New York: G & C Carvill & Co., 1838), 11–12.

32. Jacob Porter, April 12, 1810, January 29, 1810, medical journal, 1809–13, AAS.

33. Jacob Porter (1783–1845) graduated from Yale in 1803. He studied medicine under Dr. Peter Bryant, father of William Cullen Bryant.

34. John Harley Warner, *Against the System: The French Impulse in Nineteenth-Century American Medicine* (Princeton: Princeton University Press, 1998), 281.

35. Warner, *Therapeutic Perspective*, 123, 30.

36. Stephen Williams was the only physician shown as using strong cathartics more often than either mild (6%) or moderate (4%) ones. However, mild and moderate together accounted for 10 percent of his use, and strong cathartics accounted for 9 percent. Still, strong cathartics were not the bulk of his practice (see table 1.10).

37. "Costiveness" is another term for constipation.

38. John Denison Hartshorn, February 13, 1756, Journal of John Denison Hartshorn, 1754–56, Boston Medical Library, Boston (hereafter BML).

39. Thomas A. Horrocks, *Popular Print and Popular Medicine: Almanacs and Health Advice in Early America* (Amherst: University of Massachusetts Press, 2008), 67, 82.

40. Warner, *Against the Spirit of System*, 4.

41. Winchester, "Introducing Stephen West Williams," 7.

42. George Chandler, Casebook 1833, George Chandler Papers, MSS Department, Octavo folio "C," vol. 9, AAS.

43. Joseph Sargent, medical records, 1840–41, AAS.

44. New Englanders overcame seasonal limitations of dairy products and vegetables due to better storage and production by the late eighteenth and early nineteenth centuries. In the nineteenth century, vegetables began to be eaten as separate side dishes rather than simply used as flavoring for stews. Sarah F. McMahon, "A Comfortable Subsistence: The Changing Composition of Diet in Rural New England, 1620–1840," *William and Mary Quarterly* 42 (January 1985): 40–41.

45. Harvey A. Levenstein, *Revolution at the Table: The Transformation of the American Diet* (New York: Oxford University Press, 1988), 5.

46. McMahon, "A Comfortable Subsistence," 32–43.

47. Susan Williams, *Savory Suppers and Fashionable Feasts: Dining in Victorian America* (Knoxville: University of Tennessee Press, 1996), 128, 133.

48. Estes found that Aspinwall prescribed emetics 1.89 percent and Townsend 14.73 percent in the 1780s and 1790s. Estes, "Therapeutic Practice," Table XI, 316–29.
49. Gastric acids on the lining of the esophagus (throat) would have been painful, perhaps making pukes unpopular remedies.
50. Deborah Fiske to Prof. Nathan W. Fiske, Amherst, MA, October 7, 1833, Helen Hunt Jackson Papers, Special Collection, Tutt Library, Colorado College.
51. Jacob Porter, medical journal, 1809–1813, AAS.
52. By "traditional," Shorter means patients in the period of 1750 to 1850. Edward Shorter, *Bedside Manners: The Troubled History of Doctors and Patients* (New York: Simon & Schuster, 1985), 57, 61.
53. Warner, *Therapeutic Perspective*, 30.
54. Estes' data show that Aspinwall (account book from 1782 to 1795) prescribed narcotics 8.78 percent of the time, compared to using cathartics 52.33 percent of the time; Townsend (account book from 1784–1791) used narcotics 5.18 percent of the time, compared to using cathartics 21.84 percent. Though Estes' data do not show an equivalent use of opiates as cathartics, it does show that narcotics were a major class of drugs used as compared to other drug classes. See Estes, *Therapeutic Practices,* Table XI, 316–29.
55. Popular health guides such as Buchan's *Domestic Medicine* gave recipes for medicinal preparations. Recipes for anodyne balsam and paregoric elixir featured opium as their main ingredients. Presumably, Buchan and others would not have printed recipes that included ingredients unavailable to the reader. William Buchan, *Domestic Medicine: Or, the Treatise on the Prevention and Cure of Diseases By Regimen and Simple Medicines,* 11th ed. (Hartford, CT: Nathaniel Patton, 1789), 725, 766.
56. Doctor A. Seaton, "The Self-Physician," pamphlet, 1834, PAMS S441, AAS.
57. Buchan, *Domestic Medicine,* 526.
58. Warner, *Therapeutic Perspective,* 135.
59. George Chandler, medical casebook, George Chandler Papers, Mss. Dept. Octavo folio "C", vol. 9, AAS.
60. Laudanum usually referred to one of many opium tinctures. For example, laudanum liquidum was made with two ounces of opium in two pints of 100 proof alcohol allowed to stand for four days and then strained and evaporated. Estes, *Dictionary of Protopharmacology,* 113.
61. Jacob Porter, November 14, 1809, medical journal, 1809–13, AAS.
62. Ipecac induces vomiting (an emetic) and jalap irritates the small bowel (a mild cathartic). Estes, *Dictionary of Protopharmacology,* 104, 106; Joseph Sargent, August 10, 1840, medical records, 1840–41, AAS.
63. Protective eye goggles were recommended for motorists beginning in the early twentieth century. Alfred Charles William Harmsworth, *Motors and Motor-driving* (London: Longmans, Green, 1904), 73.
64. Joseph Sargent, July 31, 1840, medical records, 1840–41, AAS.
65. Although it lies outside the period of this study, White gives an unusually graphic

patient's account of surgery done in the home. Caroline Barrett White, Caroline Barrett White Papers, May 28, 1870, Octavo Volume 13, AAS.
66. Warner, *Therapeutic Perspective*, 97.
67. Daniel F. Child, 1846 diary, Daniel Franklin Child Papers, 1829–76, MHS.
68. Warner, *Therapeutic Perspective*, 97.
69. Roselyne Rey, *The History of Pain*, trans. Louise Elliott Wallace, J. A. Cadden, and S. W. Cadden (Cambridge: Harvard University Press, 1995), 126–27.
70. James Harvey Young, *The Toadstool Millionaires: A Social History of Patent Medicines in America before Federal Regulation* (Princeton: Princeton University Press, 1961), 39.
71. Young, *Toadstool Millionaires*, 32.
72. Evidence exists that physicians would prescribe medicines they considered unnecessary in order to appease their patients. I have never seen evidence that a physician deliberately gave a patient a remedy he believed had no medicinal purpose (a sugar pill, for example) in order to "trick" that patient into believing he/she would be cured by it. In modern language, I have never found evidence of a physician who knowingly prescribed a placebo to induce the placebo effect. Homeopathic physicians who gave highly diluted remedies were accused by allopathic physicians of dispensing medicines that were too diluted to have any medicinal effect. However, homeopathic physicians gave the diluted solutions believing they *did* have an effect.
73. Winchester, "Introducing Stephen West Williams," 6.
74. Jeanne Boydston discusses specialization using the shoemaker as an example. The shoemakers' labor was more and more subdivided until they became piece makers—or "nailers," "heelers," and "polishers." Jeanne Boydston, *Home and Work: Housework, Wages, and the Ideology of Labor in the Early Republic* (New York: Oxford University Press, 1990), 61.
75. Richard Harrison Shryock, *Medicine and Society in America, 1660–1860* (Ithaca, NY: Cornell University Press, 1960), 30.
76. Caleb Hopkins Snow, *A History of Boston: The Metropolis of Massachusetts, From Its Origins to the Present Period* (Boston: Abel Bowen, 1828), 4.
77. "Fifth Annual Report: Penitent Females' Refuge," *Christian Watchman*, vol. 5, no. 23 (May 15, 1824): 4.
78. Warner, *Against the Spirit*, 246.
79. "Advertisement 2—No Title," *Boston Recorder and Religious Telegraph*, October 19, 1868.
80. Warner, *Therapeutic Perspective*, 16.
81. "City Election," *Christian Watchman*, vol.5, no. 19 (April 17, 1824): 75.
82. Stephen Stowe, *Doctoring the South: Southern Physicians and Everyday Medicine in the Mid-Nineteenth Century* (Chapel Hill: University of North Carolina Press, 2004), 3.
83. Warner, *Against the Spirit*, 254.
84. Stephen Williams was also a member of the Physico-Medical Society of New York

and the Connecticut State Medical Society, an honorary member of the New York Historical Society, and a founding member of the Franklin County chapter of the Massachusetts Medical Society. "Biographical Sketch of the Late Stephen W. Williams," *Boston Medical and Surgical Journal* 53, no. 2 (1855): 29–32.
85. Stephen West Williams, January 1, 1838, October 13, 1839, medical daybook, 1836–43, PVMA.
86. Worthington Hooker, "Dissertation on the Respect Due the Medical Profession, and the Reasons That It Is Not Awarded by the Community" (Norwich, CT: J. G. Cooley Printers, 1844), 18.
87. Warner, *Therapeutic Perspective*, 134.
88. Daniel F. Child, 1846 diary, Daniel Franklin Child Papers, 1829–76, MHS.
89. Fisher served as an attending physician at the Massachusetts General Hospital from January 28, 1846, until his death in March 1850. N. I. Bowditch, *A History of the Massachusetts General Hospital* (Boston: John Wilson & Son, 1851), 410.
90. Hooker, "Dissertation on Respect," 15.
91. Jacob Porter, medical journal, 1809–13, AAS.
92. October 30, 1755, John Denison Hartshorn, Journal, BML.
93. Joseph Sargent, December 3, 1840, medical records, 1840–41, AAS.
94. George Chandler, casebook, 1833, George Chandler Papers, AAS.
95. June 12 and July 18, 1810, Jacob Porter, medical journal, AAS.
96. Sullivan, "Sanguine Practices," 220.
97. Warner, *Therapeutic Perspective*, 94.
98. Stowe, *Doctoring the South*, 155.
99. Rush was a prolific as well as quotable writer. For example, he is cited in a 1860s work as announcing, "As to nature, I would treat it in a sick chamber as I would a squalling cat—open the door and drive it out." John Spare, "Dr. Spare's Dissertation," in *Dissertation on the Part Performed by Nature and Time in the Cure of Disease; for Which Prizes Were Awarded by the Massachusetts Medical Society* (Boston: D. Clapp & Son, 1868), 97–155, as quoted in Warner, *Against the Spirit*, 282.

2. SELF-MEDICATION IN THE NINETEENTH CENTURY

1. John B. Blake, "From Buchan to Fishbein: The Literature of Domestic Medicine," in *Medicine without Doctors: Home Health Care in American History*, ed. Guenter B. Risse, Ronald L. Numbers, and Judith Walzer Leavitt (New York: Science History Publications, 1977), 25.
2. Merlin's book differs from domestic health guides such as John Wesley's *Primitive Physick* because it was a collection of recipes absent the political attacks on physicians. Blake, "From Buchan to Fishbein," 25.
3. Laurel Thatcher Ulrich, *Good Wives: Image and Reality in the Lives of Women in Northern New England, 1650–1750* (New York: Oxford University Press, 1983), 128. For more on medicinal recipes in cookbooks, see Karen Hess, *Martha Washington's Booke of Cookery* (New York: Columbia University Press, 1981), and Ann Leighton,

Early American Gardens: "For Meate or Medicine" (Boston: Houghton Mifflin, 1970).

4. Jane to Emmeline, January 20, 1842, Frederick Lewis Gay Papers, Massachusetts Historical Society, Boston (hereafter MHS).
5. Massachusetts General Hospital (MGH), medical case records, 1824–1903 [HMS b59.2], vol. 74, August to October 1836, 52.
6. Mary Gardiner Lowell, September 20, 1843, diary, vol. 81, Francis Cabot Lowell Papers, MHS.
7. The 1793 patent law did not require that an applicant demonstrate the uniqueness of his product, but it did require that the manufacturer reveal the ingredients. Thus, most nostrum makers found other ways to protect their products, such as patenting a distinctive shape or color of the container, or the method of composition. James Harvey Young, *The Toadstool Millionaires: A Social History of Patent Medicines in America before Federal Regulation* (Princeton: Princeton University Press, 1961), 40. By the end of the American Revolution there were 43 weekly papers. The first daily newspaper appeared in 1784, and by 1800 there were 20 daily papers; in 1860 there were 400. See William H. Helfand, "Advertising Health to the People," in *"Every Man His Own Doctor": Popular Medicine in Early America,* ed. William Helfand and Charles Rosenberg (Philadelphia: The Library Company of Philadelphia, 1998), 33, and Young, *Toadstool Millionaires,* 39.
8. Young, *Toadstool Millionaires,* 7.
9. Helfand, "Advertising Health," 27.
10. Young, *Toadstool Millionaires,* 21.
11. Advertisement, "Dr. Relf's Botanical Drops," *Boston Gazette,* May 11, 1820, American Antiquarian Society, Worcester, MA (hereafter AAS).
12. MGH, medical case records, vol. 144, May to August 1848, 56. J. Worth Estes, *Dictionary of Protopharmacology: Therapeutic Practices, 1700–1850* (Canton, MA: Science History Publications, 1990), 47.
13. Jacob Porter, *Medical Journal, 1809–13,* AAS.
14. Ann Leighton, *American Gardens of the Nineteenth Century: "For Comfort and Affluence"* (Amherst: University of Massachusetts Press, 1987), 16.
15. James H. Stuart to Margaret S. Forster, April 28, 1846, Forster Family Letters, 1819–87, Francis C. Wood Institute for the History of Medicine, Philadelphia (hereafter Wood).
16. Worthington Hooker, *Dissertation on the Respect Due the Medical Profession, and the Reasons That It Is Not Awarded by the Community* (Norwich, CT: J. G. Cooley Printer, 1844), 7.
17. Ambrose Seaton, *The Self-Physician, or Newly Invented Medicine Chest, for Family, Sea or Plantation Use* (Boston, 1834), AAS.
18. It is unclear whether Gordak graduated from medical school, served an apprenticeship, or was a self-styled practitioner.
19. "Dr. Gordak's Jelly of Pomegranate and Peruvian Pills," Pamphlets (PAMS G661 Dr 1831), AAS. Costiveness refers to constipation; scrofula to tuberculosis of the lymph

nodes, especially in the neck; erysipelas to a disease associated with inflammation of the skin. Tetters referred to various skin diseases such as eczema or psoriasis.
20. The testimony was dated November 11, 1837. "Gordak's Jelly."
21. Young, *Toadstool Millionaires*, 187–88.
22. Ibid., 137, 139.
23. In advertisements for Dr. Herrick's products, his credentials are listed thus: "DR. HERRICK, THE INVENTOR of these Pills, is a regularly educated physician; a man of years, experience and standing, a pupil and graduate of the University of Massachusetts, who has enjoyed years of successful practice, and is well calculated to adopt remedies for the successful cure of a multitude of diseases which afflict mankind." *Terrific Fight with Savages; A Reminiscence of Border Life: To Which Is Added a Guide to Health, Wealth and Happiness* (Albany, NY: Dr. Herrick & Brothers, Chemists, 1858), 8.
24. Herrick, *Terrific Fight with Savages*, 1–31. Dr. Edward Norman was born in Hudson, NY, in 1806; he removed to North Adams in 1830 and opened the first drug store there, selling out in 1859 to W. H. Griswold and a Dr. Lawrence. Norman married Miss L. M. Putnam, a great-granddaughter of General Israel Putnam, by whom he had two children. He died on May 28, 1874. See "History of North Adams," "Dr. Edward Norman," www.dunhamwilcox.net/ma/north_adams_ma.htm.
25. MGH, medical case records, vol. 64, May 23, 1835, 248.
26. MGH, medical case records, vol. 134, April 29, 1847, 3.
27. For more information on methodology and the exact dates of volume sampled of the records of MGH data, see appendix E.
28. See appendix E for further information on the methodology used.
29. In 1822, MGH provided around 22 percent of its patients with totally free care. After 1830, circa 40 percent of patients did not pay any fee. Leonard K. Eaton, *New England Hospitals, 1790–1833* (Ann Arbor: University of Michigan Press, 1957), 104–6, 189; Charles E. Rosenberg, *The Care of Strangers: The Rise of America's Hospital System* (New York: Basic Books, 1987), 21.
30. This mortality rate is higher than comparative deaths in Ireland. From May 14, 1804, to Jan. 5, 1816, Cork Street Fever Hospital of Dublin reported 20, 278 patients with typhus. In 1805, the hospital reported the highest mortality rate at 10 percent, with an average of 7 percent. The house physicians at MGH in the 1830s may have recorded incidences of typhoid fever as typhus fever. Categorized as a distinct fever in 1829, typhoid often was documented as typhus into the mid-nineteenth century. Elisha Bartlett wrote that "in New England it [typhoid] has been generally known under the name of typhus or typhus fever; and by a great majority of practitioners it still continues to be so designated." Elisha Bartlett, *History, Diagnosis, and Treatment of Typhus and Typhoid Fevers; with an Essay on the Diagnosis of Bilious Remittent and of Yellow Fever* (Philadelphia: Lea & Blanchard, 1842), 257, 3.
31. Rosenberg, *Care of Strangers*, 26, 31. MGH, medical case records, vol. 74, September 1, 1836, 42.

32. James Parkinson, MD, *Medical Admonitions to Families, Respecting the Preservation of Health, and the Treatment of the Sick* (Portsmouth, NH: N. W. & W. Pierce, 1803), 6, 7, 76.
33. Private practitioners showed similar high rates of use of cathartics (20–36% range, with the exception of Snow at 14%). See chapter 1.
34. Semiskilled and service workers constituted the largest growing segment of patients that entered MGH. This will be discussed in chapter 3.
35. Lewis Merlin, *The Treasure of Health, or, A Wonderful Collection of the Most Valuable Secrets in Medicine* (Philadelphia: Printed for the society, 1819), 253–55. Lydia Maria Child, *The American Frugal Housewife, Dedicated to Those Who Are Not Afraid of Economy* (Boston: Carter, Hendee & Co., 1833), 27.
36. Eaton, *New England Hospitals*, 178.
37. Edward Shorter, *Bedside Manners: The Troubled History of Doctors and Patients* (New York: Simon & Schuster, 1985), 61. Shorter defines the traditional patient as one who was ill from 1750 to 1850 and uses the descriptive "alternative healers" differently than I have (see below, page 170, note 37). He includes midwives and lay healers in the category of "alternative."
38. Daniel F. Child, February 3 and 5, 1848, diary, Daniel Franklin Child Papers, 1829–76, MHS.
39. MGH, medical case records, vol. 134, April 1, 1847, 167.
40. Calomel was a strong cathartic made with mercury. Jalap still is a mild cathartic. Pinkroot and senna were common ingredients prescribed by physicians. Pinkroot refers to Carolina pinkroot, or spigelia, which is an anthelmintic to remove worms from the intestinal canal. Senna was a cathartic. See Estes, *Dictionary of Protopharmacology*, 34, 106, 181, 176.
41. Jacob Porter, November 14, 1809, medical journal, 1809–13, AAS. Also see passages from December 7, December 11 and December 14, 1809.
42. Chandler Robbins, 1768 interleaved almanac, 3, P-363, reel 7.12, MHS.
43. Hugh Lenox Hodge 1796–1873, ledger, box 1, Wood, as paraphrased from the works of John Gregory, *Lectures on the Duty and Qualifications of a Physician* (London, 1772).
44. As stipulated in the Introduction, "unorthodox" refers to healers and practitioners who were not "trained" by a medical school or through apprenticeship and/or were not considered by the bulk of practitioners as members of their profession. Thus, "unorthodox" includes midwives, Indian healers, bonesetters, and Thomasonians, as well as alternative healers such as homeopaths and eclectics.
45. Joseph Sargent, August 20, 1840, medical records, 1840–41, AAS.
46. Rebecca Packard to Asa Packard, February 12, 1830, Packard Family Papers, AAS.
47. The word "quack" can be dated to 1543, according to the Oxford English Dictionary. It is a shortened form of the Dutch word *Kwaksalver* or *quacksalver*, a person who cures with home remedies. Used as a noun by 1638, "quack" took on the derogatory meaning of a person who dishonestly claims to have medical or surgical expertise. As a verb, "quacking" can mean to pretend to have medical or surgical skills, or to

dabble ignorantly in medicine (tracing back to 1650). "Quacksalver," *OED*, 2nd ed., vol. 12 (Oxford: Clarendon Press, 1989), 953.

48. Mrs. Shattuck often wrote in her husband's journal. George C. Shattuck, Jr., July 29, 1840, dairy 1834–42, George Shattuck Jr. Papers, MHS.

49. For information on Thomsonian and homeopathic medicine, see chapter 1, n. 4. Eclectics utilized different aspects of the "pathies." In other words, they combined treatments from several different therapeutic camps. Hydropathy, or the Water Cure, reached the height of its popularity from 1840 to 1870. Practitioners of it believed there were two causes of disease: lack of vitality and violations of hygienic laws. For more information, see Norman Gevitz, ed., *Other Healers: Unorthodox Medicine in America* (Baltimore: Johns Hopkins University Press, 1988).

50. Worthington Hooker, *The Treatment Due from the Medical Profession, to Physicians Who Become Homeopathic Practitioners* (Norwich, CT: John G. Cooley, 1852), 5–6 (emphasis in original). Hooker uses the term "empiric" synonymously with "quack." As John H. Warner explains, "Nineteenth-century American physicians had inherited a long-established equation of the empiric and the quack." The use of "empiric" as a condemnatory term was inherited from seventeenth-century England. However, as the nineteenth century proceeded, empiricism enjoyed a comeback. The approach, Warner states, was considered "essential to the 'scientific physician.'" In other words, empiricism persisted as a negative professional term but increasingly emerged as a positive methodological term. "This multiplicity of meanings for the two words most central to the ongoing reassessment of therapeutic knowledge confused programmatic statements and greatly clouded discussion." Therapeutics based on empiricism relied on experience or, in the case of the nineteenth century, scientific observation, and rationalism depended on theory. John Harley Warner, *Therapeutic Perspectives: The Medical Practice, Knowledge and Identity in America, 1820–1885* (Princeton: Princeton University Press, 1997), 44–45.

51. James H. Stuart to Margaret S. Forster, March 12, 1849, letter, Forster Family Papers, 1819–87, Wood. Stuart's use of the word "august" suggests that he was somewhat skeptical of his aunt's and uncle's choice.

52. Elizabeth P. Peabody, *Memorial of Dr. William Wesselhöft* (Boston: Nathaniel C. Peabody, 1859), 25, 34.

53. MGH, medical case records, vol. 74, September 9, 1836, 68; vol. 134, March 18, 1847, 115; and vol. 154, August 6, 1849, 192.

54. MGH, medical case records, vol. 44, September 26, 1831, 152 and September 30, 1831, 178.

3. MONEY AND MEDICINE

1. Ben Mutschler, "Illness in the 'Social Credit' and 'Money' Economies of Eighteenth-Century New England," in *Medicine and the Market in England and Its Colonies, c. 1450–c. 1850*, ed. Mark S. R. Jenner and Patrick Wallis (New York: Palgrave

Macmillan, 2007), 177. Ben Mutschler, "The Province of Affliction: Illness in New England, 1690–1820" (PhD diss., Columbia University, 2000), 57.
2. Christopher Clark, *The Roots of Rural Capitalism: Western Massachusetts, 1780–1860* (Ithaca, NY: Cornell University Press, 1990), 69, 33.
3. Martin Bruegel, *Farm, Shop, Landing: The Rise of a Market Society in the Hudson Valley, 1780–1860* (Durham, NC: Duke University Press, 2002), 4; Mark S. R. Jenner and Patrick Wallis, "The Medical Marketplace," in *Medicine and the Market in England and Its Colonies, c. 1450–c. 1850* (New York: Palgrave Macmillan, 2007), 8.
4. Clark, *Roots of Rural Capitalism*, 60. Naomi R. Lamoreaux claims that the moral-economy historians, a category in which Clark is included, depict a dichotomy between precapitalist farmers and merchants that does not exist. She demonstrates through rural merchant account books that merchants were constrained by family and community as well. The "rational economic man" should be abandoned for a more neoclassical theory that treats "*firms* as profit-maximizing entities" and "holds that *individuals* maximize utility." Naomi R. Lamoreaux, "Rethinking the Transition to Capitalism in the Early American Northeast," *Journal of American History* 90 (September 2003): 449.
5. Clark, *Roots of Rural Capitalism*, 12, 31, 197.
6. Ibid., 197.
7. Josiah Brigham, account book, 1785–91, American Antiquarian Society, Worcester, MA (hereafter AAS).
8. Edward Flint, medical ledger, 1766–90, AAS.
9. Moses Mosman, account books, 1783–1820, AAS.
10. Clark, *Roots of Rural Capitalism*, 35.
11. See Gamaliel Bradford, daybook, no. 1, 1819–39, Francis C. Wood Institute, College of Physicians, Philadelphia (hereafter Wood); George S. Shattuck, Jr., daybook, 1833–36, Francis A. Countway Library of Medicine, Boston (hereafter Countway); and Caleb H. Snow, account books, 1826–28, Caleb H. Snow Papers, Massachusetts. Historical Society, Boston (MHS).
12. By cash payment, I mean banknotes, hard coins, or federally minted paper currency. Banknotes served as a promise of payment in an equivalent amount of gold and silver coin when presented at the bank. In the period from the American Revolution up to the Civil War, there was little "hard" money circulating; banks provided a medium of exchange. The term "note" signifies promissory notes, IOUs, and notes of hand (I use the terms interchangeably), a paper signed by both parties in which the debtor agreed to make some form of payment by a specified date. Stephen Mihm, *A Nation of Counterfeiters: Capitalists, Con Men, and the Making of the United States* (Cambridge: Harvard University Press, 2007), 3.
13. For methodology, see appendix E.
14. Nathaniel Saltonstall, ledger, 1769–83, Nathaniel Saltonstall Papers, 1746–1815, MHS.
15. On several occasions he actually writes out the note in his 1783–1815 ledger. For examples, see notes dated October 25, 1802, from John Chickering and February 17, 1815, from Joel Harriman.

16. Only twice did Dr. Snow receive payment in kind. Snow, account book, 1826–28, MHS.
17. See also Dr. John Green II, account books, Green Family of Worcester, MA. Papers, 1764–1908, AAS.
18. Mihm, *Nation of Counterfeiters*, 11–12. Bruegel, *Farm, Shop, Landing*, 219–20.
19. Clark, *Roots of Rural Capitalism*, 225.
20. If you compare Flint's ledger from 1766–90 to his ledger from 1795–1816, the amount of notes clearly increases. See table 3.2.
21. Clark, *Roots of Rural Capitalism*, 124, 36, 37.
22. Ibid., 196.
23. William S. Williams, account books, vol. 1, 1787–1828, and vol. 2, 1807–28, Pocumtuck Valley Memorial Association, Deerfield, Massachusetts (hereafter PMVA).
24. Amos A. Taylor, account book, 1828–48, PVMA. Out of 281 entries analyzed (first 90 pages), 122 were in cash (43%), 113 in goods (40%), and 46 in notes (16%). Steven Stowe found similar patterns in the rural South: "Daybooks all through the [nineteenth] century reveal a thick texture of in-kind exchange; patients and doctors constantly weighed a medical procedure—pulling a tooth—against, say, a basket of fruit." Steven M. Stowe, *Doctoring the South: Southern Physicians and Everyday Medicine in the Mid-Nineteenth Century* (Chapel Hill: University of North Carolina Press, 2004), 112.
25. See note 12 above for definitions. Mihm, *Nation of Counterfeiters*, 3.
26. Clark, *Roots of Rural Capitalism*, 71.
27. For a few examples see entries July 28, 1836, February 24, 1837, July 17, 1837, and June 14, 1838, in Stephen West Williams, July 18, 1836–September 19, 1843, daybook, PVMA. James Harvey Young, *The Toadstool Millionaires: A Social History of Patent Medicines in America before Federal Regulation* (Princeton: Princeton University Press, 1961), 32.
28. Zadok Howe, "Dr. Howe's Discourse on Quackery," *Boston Medical and Surgical Journal* (hereafter *BSMJ*) 11, no. 3 (August 27, 1834): 47; Gamma, "Medical Reflections.—no. i," *BSMJ* 11, no. 8 (October 1, 1834): 130.
29. The other three types of patients are those who never intended to pay; those who can and will pay "on compulsion"; and, the most enviable of patients, those of the "redeeming class" who "pay promptly, liberally, and cheerfully." "Collection of Medical Debts," *BSMJ* 33, no. 10 (October 8, 1845): 201. In fact, "the fundamental motivations in founding America's first hospitals was an unquestioned distinction between the worthy and unworthy poor, between the prudent and industrious objects of benign stewardship and those less deserving Americans whose own failings justified their almshouse incarceration." Charles E. Rosenberg, *In the Care of Strangers: The Rise of the American Hospital System* (New York: Basic Books, 1987), 19.
30. Caleb H. Snow, 1826 account book, Caleb H. Snow Papers, MHS.
31. John George Metcalf, medical ledger, 1844–83, Wood.

32. Lamoreaux, "Rethinking the Transition," 457.
33. Barry Hankins, *The Second Great Awakening and the Transcendentalists* (Westport, CT: Greenwood Press, 2004), 3.
34. "Cheating Physicians Out of their Dues," *BSMJ* 33, no. 8 (September 24, 1845): 162.
35. "Collection of Medical Debts," *BSMJ* 33, no. 10 (October 8, 1845): 201.
36. "Profits of a Medical Practice," *BSMJ* 36, no. 10 (April 7, 1847): 203.
37. I am distinguishing between choices among irregulars and alternative healers, both of whom fall under the category of unorthodox. Irregular healers did not offer any substantially new therapies or treatments; they specialized as eye doctors, cancer doctors, and bone setters, or they touted "cures" that claimed to rid patients of a variety of ailments. Alternative healers of the nineteenth century, such as electric doctors, hydropaths, and homeopaths, offered "new" treatments that differed in some form from those of regular practice and founded their authority on science. In fact, many homeopaths and hydropaths were MDs. Thomsonians fall under the category of irregulars, because they did not offer anything substantially new in therapeutics but offered every man the chance to be his own physician. Norman Gevitz, ed., *Other Healers: Unorthodox Medicine in America* (Baltimore: Johns Hopkins University Press, 1988), 1–28.
38. Stowe, *Doctoring the South,* 122.
39. J. F. Skinner, "Domestic Medicine," *BSMJ* 40, no. 16 (May 23, 1849): 2. J. L. Chandler, "Nostrum Trade," *BSMJ* 38, no. 4 (February 23, 1848): 73.
40. Charles Rosenberg, "And Heal the Sick: The Hospital and the Patient in the 19th Century," *Journal of Social History* 10 (Summer 1977), 431. Charles Rosenberg, *The Care of Strangers: The Rise of America's Hospital System* (New York: Basic Books), 23.
41. By 1830, an annual subscription drive meant that 40 percent of patients were provided free care. Eaton, *New England Hospitals,* 104; Rosenberg, *Care of Strangers,* 19, 23.
42. Charles Rosenberg demonstrated that the hospital in the first half of the nineteenth century was not an acute-care facility but a place where patients who had nowhere else to go for medical treatment came. Often these patients surrendered their autonomy for the security of room and board as well as medical treatment. See chapter 1, "To Heal the Sick: The Antebellum Hospital and Society," in Rosenberg, *Care of Strangers.*
43. The Boston dispensary opened in 1796.
44. Abbie Dunks, "The Boston Dispensary, 1796–1962," *New England Journal of Medicine* 266 (January 1962): 29. Eaton, *New England Hospitals,* 187.
45. Frances Byerly Parkes, *Domestic Duties: or, Instructions to Young Married Ladies, On the Management of Their Households, and the Regulation of Their Conduct in the Various Relations and Duties of Married Life* (New York: J. & J. Harper, 1828), 112. This was a first American edition adapted for American audiences from a London third edition. The book enjoyed many reprintings and was considered one of the leading domestic advice manuals in the late 1820s. Carolyn L. Karcher, *The First Woman in the Republic: A Cultural Biography of Lydia Maria Child* (Durham, NC: Duke University Press, 1994), 128.

46. MGH, medical case records, 1824–1903 [HMS b59.2], vol. 3, May 23, 1823, 54.
47. The use of the word "stupid" most likely referred to the patient's impaired mental state rather than to a lack of intelligence. MGH, medical case records, vol. 154, August 14, 1849, 222.
48. For example, from the 1835, 1836, 1837, and 1839 sampled volumes, 129 new patients were recorded as married, single, or widowed. Thirty-one percent were single males and 29 percent single females. In the same volumes, widowed women comprised 5 percent of the total.
49. MGH, medical case records, vol. 13, December 1, 1825, 242.
50. N. I. Bowditch, *A History of the Massachusetts General Hospital* (Boston: J. Wilson & Son, 1851), 6–7.
51. A breakdown of the ages of patients admitted to MGH is as follows: 1820–29 mean age was 29.96 out of a total of 222; 1830–39 mean age was 27.76 out of a total of 265; and 1840–49 mean age was 30.31 out of a total of 257. Year range represents range of sampled volumes; see appendix E.
52. MGH, medical case records, vol. 24, August 16, 1827, 109.

4. PATIENT EXPECTATIONS AND RELIGIOUS BELIEFS

1. Louisa Jane Trumbull, February 7, 1883, diary, Trumbull Family Papers, 1773–1903, Octavo vol. 16, American Antiquarian Society, Worcester, MA (AAS).
2. Robert Fuller, *Alternative Medicine and American Religious Life* (New York: Oxford University Press, 1989), 60–65; Roselyn Rey, *The History of Pain,* trans. Louise Elliot Wallace, J. A. Cadden, and S. W. Cadden (Cambridge: Harvard University Press, 1995), 98; Elaine Forman Crane, "'I Have Suffer'd So Much': The Defining Force of Pain in Early America," in *Through a Glass Darkly: Reflection on Personal Identity in Early America,* ed. Ronald Hoffman, Mechel Sobel, and Fredrika J. Teute (Chapel Hill: University of North Carolina University Press, 1997), 375; and Donald Caton, MD, "The Secularization of Pain," *Anesthesiology* 62 (1985): 495–97.
3. This study does not substantially discuss the topics of surgery or epidemics but addresses common ailments.
4. The *OED* traces two meanings of the word "cure"—"the treatment of disease, or of a patient" and "successful medical treatment; the action or process of healing a wound, a disease, or a sick person; restoration of health"—back to the fourteenth century; "Cure," in *Oxford English Dictionary* (New York: Oxford University Press, 2010), 428. I argue that the former usage was more common until the late eighteenth and early nineteenth centuries, when the latter meaning seems to have dominated.
5. Franklin Bowditch Dexter, *Yale Biographies and Annals,* vol. 2 (New York: Henry Holt, 1885), 328–30.
6. He practiced medicine among his parishioners, but does not appear to have treated his father. Justus Forward, February 10 and March 24, 1776, Justus Forward

Diaries, 1762–97, AAS (hereafter Justus Forward diary). For more on the tradition of preacher-physician, see Patricia A. Watson, *The Angelical Conjunction: The Preacher-Physicians of Colonial New England* (Knoxville: University of Tennessee Press, 1991).
7. Justus Forward diary, April 30, 1766.
8. Daniel White Wells and Reuben Field Wells, *A History of Hatfield, Massachusetts* (Springfield, MA: F. C. H. Gibbons, 1910), 205–7.
9. Anna Sophia (Parkman) Brigham to Josiah Brigham, June 8, 1783, Parkman Family Papers, AAS.
10. John Syng Dorsey, ledger vol. 1, John Syng Dorsey Ledgers, 1804–17, Wood.
11. Hugh Lenox Hodge 1796–1873, ledger, box 1, Wood, as paraphrased from John Gregory, *Lectures and Duties on the Qualifications of a Physician* (Philadelphia: M. Carey & Son, 1817), 22. Hodge references other physician-authors such as Benjamin Rush in a commonplace book.
12. Ben Mutschler, "The Province of Affliction: Illness in New England, 1690–1820" (PhD diss., Columbia University, 2000), 39–41. Although the expression in letters "I hope this finds you well" is still in use, Mutschler demonstrates the prevalence of these expressions by citing many examples in eighteenth-century diaries in which the author described having found someone well or sick.
13. Mary Lindemann arrives at a different conclusion in her analysis of eighteenth-century German patients: "The long-term quests of such patients, as they moved from healer to healer, convincingly show that they indeed pursued cures. It has often been argued that early modern people did not really expect healers to banish their ailments completely, hoping rather to find alleviation of pain, to confirm their own diagnosis, or to understand their prognosis. But in the cases analyzed here, it is plain that patients primarily aspired to a restoration of health." Mary Lindemann, *Health and Healing in Eighteenth-Century Germany* (Baltimore: Johns Hopkins University Press, 1996), 351. The eighteenth-century English and German medical practices appear more like the medical practices of nineteenth-century America.
14. John Harley Warner, *The Therapeutic Perspective: Medical Practice, Knowledge and Identity in America, 1820–1885* (Princeton: Princeton University Press, 1997), 92.
15. *The World of Hannah Heaton: The Diary of an Eighteenth-Century New England Farm Woman*, ed. Barbara E. Lacey (DeKalb: Northern Illinois University Press, 2003), 227.
16. Transcript of the Diary of Experience (Wight) Richardson, 1728–82, ed. Ellen Glueck and Thelma Ernst, MHS.
17. Marla R. Miller, "'My Part Alone': The World of Rebecca Dickinson, 1787–1802," *New England Quarterly* 71 (September 1998): 351.
18. Mutschler, "Province of Affliction," 36.
19. See chapter 2 for more information on advertisements of itinerant practitioners and their promises of cure.
20. Crane, "I Have Suffer'd So Much," 375.

21. Jacob Porter, medical journal, October 30 and November 18, 1809, AAS.
22. Perhaps he attempted to treat himself but was unsuccessful. Self-treatment is discussed in chapter 2.
23. Porter, journal, March 23, 1810, AAS.
24. See Porter, journal, March 23, 28, 31 and April 10, 17, 28, 1810, AAS, for records of relief, and April 12 and 20 for notations of a relapse of the headaches.
25. James Jackson, Sr., to James Jackson, Jr., Boston, March 20, 1833, Jackson Papers, Countway.
26. Louisa Adams Park, diary, July 10, 1848, Park Family Papers, 1800–90, inscription by Dr. Park, AAS.
27. Park diary, May 2, 1801, AAS. Scrofula was a swelling in the lymph nodes, especially those of the neck. Modern medicine understands the term to indicate primary tuberculosis in the lymph nodes.
28. Park diary, May 2, 1801, AAS.
29. Ibid.
30. Cures were often promised by "patent" medicines advertised in newspapers. Perhaps patients had become weary of empty promises and physicians leery of using words that might associate them with quackery. The subjects of proprietary medicines and self-medication are addressed in chapter 2.
31. Carl von Rokitansky and Rudolf Virchow in Germany are credited with the emergence of cell and organ pathology. Experiments showing links between brain-lesion clinical work were done in Edinburgh by John Abercrombie and Richard Bright. Caton, "The Secularization of Pain," 497.
32. Crane, "I Have Suffer'd So Much." 372.
33. I borrow Charles D. Cashdollar's definition of providence as referring to the manner in which God operates in the world, with respect to both man and nature. Charles D. Cashdollar, "The Social Implications of the Doctrine of Divine Providence: A Nineteenth-Century Debate in American Theology," *Harvard Theological Review* 71 (July–October 1978): 266.
34. Cashdollar, "Social Implications," 271–72.
35. Shelia M. Rothman, *Living in the Shadow of Death: Tuberculosis and the Social Experience of Illness in American History* (New York: Basic Books, 1994), 109.
36. "Consumption" referred to a lung disease we now call tuberculosis. During most of the nineteenth century, physicians believed that consumption was hereditary rather than contagious.
37. Deborah Vinal Fiske, as quoted in Rothman, *Living in the Shadow of Death,* 109.
38. Deborah Vinal Fiske to Nathan W. Fiske, October 7, 1833, Helen Hunt Jackson Papers, Special Collections, Tutt Library, Colorado College (hereafter HHJ).
39. Deborah Vinal Fiske to Nathan W. Fiske, October 9, 1833, HHJ.
40. Rothman, *Living in the Shadow of Death,* 105, 81–83 and chap. 7.
41. Mark A. Noll, *America's God: From Jonathan Edwards to Abraham Lincoln* (New York: Oxford University Press, 2003), 287.
42. Conrad Wright, "Institutional Reconstruction in the Unitarian Controversy," in

American Unitarianism, 1805–1865, ed. Conrad Edick Wright (Boston: Northeastern University Press, 1989), 3–11.
43. Daniel Walker Howe, *The Unitarian Conscience: Harvard Moral Philosophy, 1805–1861* (Cambridge: Harvard University Press, 1970), 4.
44. Noll, *America's God,* 140. Gary Dorrien, *The Making of American Liberal Theology: Imagining Progressive Religion, 1805–1900* (Louisville, KY: Westminster John Knox Press, 2001), 1–4, 19. Conrad Wright, *The Beginnings of Unitarianism in America* (Boston: Beacon Press, 1955), 48–49.
45. William Ellery Channing, "Unitarian Christianity," in *William Ellery Channing: Selected Writings,* ed. David Robinson (New York: Paulist Press, 1985), 89, 94, 77.
46. Noll, *America's God,* 139.
47. Unitarians extended this belief in self-improvement to society. They had a specific program of reform in their involvement in domestic missions. For example, the Benevolent Fraternity of Unitarians and Universalist churches began in 1825 to provide aid to the poor and immigrants in Boston. Yet, the majority of Unitarians were not active in the antislavery movement. Channing came out in support of abolition but admitted that most Unitarians showed little interest in the issue. In fact, Channing's church, Federal Street Church, refused to host either preachers who gave antislavery sermons or the convention of the New England Anti-Slavery Convention in 1835. Conrad Wright argues that dominant representation of the mercantile elites among the Unitarian congregation might account for this lack of interest: to incite national division over slavery would interrupt their commercial interests. Spencer Lavan and George Huntston Williams, "The Unitarian and Universalist Traditions," in *Caring and Curing: Health and Medicine in the Western Religious Traditions,* ed. Ronald L. Numbers and Darrel W. Amundsen (Baltimore: Johns Hopkins University Press, 1998), 364. Wright, ed., *American Unitarianism,* 192–93.
48. Child, diaries, November 26, 1839, February 18, 1840, and February 13, 1848, Child Papers, MHS.
49. Child, diaries, November 6, 1847 and January 31, 1846, MHS.
50. Child, diaries 1843 and 1847, January 6, 1843 and December 7, 1847, Daniel Franklin Child Papers, 1829–76, MHS. For other examples of attendance at medical lectures, see November 30, 1847, December 10, 1847, and October 16, 1848.
51. Child, diaries, April 23, 1849, MHS.
52. In the late eighteenth century, Luigi Galvani of Bologna initially experimented with electricity and its effects on neuromuscular tissue after dissecting a frog on a table that accidently rested on an electrical machine: one of his students had happened to touch the dead frog's leg with a charged dissecting knife, causing the leg to contract. By the early nineteenth century, the debate among scientists was whether there existed an "electric fluid" or "galvanic fluid" that served as a "principal agent in the vital process of each organ" that could become unbalanced and cause illnesses. Despite the questionable conclusion, many itinerant doctors emerged who promised to cure ailments such as paralysis, pain, insanity, and many

other afflictions through the use of galvanic batteries or other apparatuses. Carl J. Pfeiffer, *The Art and Practice of Western Medicine in the Early Nineteenth Century* (Jefferson, NC: McFarland, 1985), 19, 25, 38–40.
53. Child, dairies, June 3–19, 1848, December 16–27, 1848, and August 24, 1849, MHS. Dr. William Wesselhoeft, who is referred to here, was the brother of Robert Wesselhoeft, one of the pioneers of hydropathy or water-cure treatments in the United States. John S. Haller, Jr., *The History of American Homeopathy: The Academic Years, 1820–1935* (New York: Pharmaceutical Products Press, 2005), 46. For more information on Paige's practice, see Dr. A. Paige, *The Electropathic Guide Devoted to Electricity and Its Medical Application* (Boston: Damrell & Moore, 1849), and Brenda Himrich and Stewart Thornley, *Electrifying Medicine: How Electricity Sparked a Medical Revolution* (Minneapolis: Lerner Publishing, 1995). For biographical information on Adams, see Charles N. Peabody, *Zab: Brevet Major Zabdiel Boylston Adams, 1829–1902, Physician of Boston and Framingham* (Boston: Francis C. Countway Library of Medicine, 1984); and on Wesselhoeft, see Elizabeth A. Peabody, *Memorial of Dr. William Wesselhöft* (Boston: Nathaniel C. Peabody, 1859).
54. Child, Diaries, August 23, 1849, MHS.
55. See insert written by Jessie Rodriquez, 1982 in the folder of Lucy Chase, diary October 19, 1841–March 3, 1842, Chase Family Papers, AAS.
56. Chase diary, April 12, 1842.
57. Chase diary, September 22 and 23, 1842.
58. S. E. D. Short, "Physicians, Science, and Status: Issues in the Professionalization of Anglo-American Medicine in the Nineteenth Century," *Medical History* 27 (1983): 64.
59. For a discussion on preachers' effects on religious scripts and their reception by the congregations, see Erik R. Seeman, *Pious Persuasions: Laity and Clergy in Eighteenth-Century New England* (Baltimore: Johns Hopkins University Press, 1999).
60. Mary Heath, November 1, 1824, August 5–December 2, 1824, diary, Heath Family Papers, MHS (hereafter Mary Heath dairy).
61. Mary Heath diary, November 7, 1824.
62. Ibid., November 21, 1824.
63. Ibid., July 27, 1824, April 11–April 30, 1824.
64. *The Massachusetts Medical Society, Medical Communications* lists Charles Wild of Brookline as a member of the Massachusetts Medical Society, a society of orthodox physicians. "Other 3—No Title," *Massachusetts Medical Society, Medical Communications (1790–1913)*, vol. 4 (Boston: American Periodicals Series II, 1829), a1. Interestingly, Dr. Wild began "investigating homoeopathy" in the year 1840. *History of Homoeopathy and Its Institutions in America*, ed. William Harvey King, vol. 1 (New York: Lewis Publishing, 1905), 216.
65. McGovern does state that the church eventually united under Unitarianism. James R. McGovern, *Yankee Family* (New Orleans, LA: Polyanthos, 1975), 33–35.
66. Philip F. Gura, *American Transcendentalism: A History* (New York: Hill & Wang, 2007), 14.

· NOTES TO PAGES 82–84 ·

67. Ralph Waldo Emerson, "Harvard Divinity School Address," in *American Religions: A Documentary History*, ed. R. Marie Griffith (New York: Oxford University Press, 2008), 173–74.
68. Parker disagreed with Emerson on the practical application of transcendentalism, believing that he overemphasized self-reliance. God was not just part of us, but what man needed to become whole, according to Parker. One way to connect with God was to become selflessly devoted to social reform. Emerson criticized all the associations for social reform by arguing that they served merely as distractions from the inner spiritual work that needed to be done; a person must undergo an inner spiritual transformation before joining similarly enlightened people to work on the ills of the outer world. Gura, *American Transcendentalism*, 210–11, 218.
69. Cashdollar, "Social Implications," 277.
70. Megan Marshall, *The Peabody Sisters: Three Women Who Ignited American Romanticism* (New York: Houghton Mifflin, 2006), 463n4. Also see Bruce A. Ronda, *Elizabeth Palmer Peabody: A Reformer on Her Own Terms* (Cambridge: Harvard University Press, 1999).
71. Caroline Healey Dall, *Daughter of Boston: The Extraordinary Diary of a Nineteenth-Century Woman*, ed. Helen R. Deese (Boston: Beacon Press, 2005), xvi.
72. Ibid., 127.
73. Ibid., 189.
74. Most regular physicians rejected homeopathy. Walter Channing's biographer described Channing's attitude toward homeopathy as scathing; "The notion that infinitesimal doses of like substances can cure disease was completely antithetical to every theory of regular medicine as well as common sense, and he had absolutely no patience with it." Amalie M. Kass, *Midwifery and Medicine in Boston, Walter Channing, MD, 1786–1876* (Boston: Northeastern University Press, 2002), 235. Dr. William Wesselhoeft is credited with creating interest in homeopathy in Boston beginning in 1842.
75. Fuller, *Alternative Medicine*, 26.
76. Anne Taylor Kirschmann, *A Vital Force: Women in American Homeopathy* (New Brunswick, NJ: Rutgers University Press, 2004), 31.
77. Elisabeth Alcott died from her illness in 1858. A. Bronson Alcott, *Letters of A. Bronson Alcott*, ed. Richard L. Hernstadt (Ames: Iowa University Press, 1969), 254. Dr. Christian F. Geist immigrated from Germany in 1835, studied under homeopathic physician Robert Wesselhoeft, and practiced mostly in Boston. William Harvey King, *History of Homoeopathy*, vol. 1 (New York and Chicago: Lewis Publishing, 1905), 227.
78. Louisa May Alcott has been described by historian Anne Kirschmann as having had a long-standing relationship with homeopathic doctor Conrad Wesselhoeft. Kirschmann, *A Vital Force*, 32.
79. A. Bronson Alcott, *Letters*, 206, 208. Dr. Russell Trall (1812–77) trained in allopathic medicine, dabbled in homeopathic medicine, and then settled into practice as a hygieno-therapist, a practitioner who emphasized preventive medicine through cold baths, exercise, and diet. Kirschmann, *A Vital Force*, 90.

80. A. Bronson Alcott, *Letters*, 159. Louisa May Alcott, *The Selected Letters of Louisa May Alcott*, ed. Joel Myerson and Daniel Shealy (Boston: Little, Brown, 1987), 306, 285–86, 287–88. For more on the mind cure, see Fuller, *Alternative Medicine*, 60–65.
81. Noll, *America's God*, 176.
82. Howe, *Unitarian Conscience*, 163–64.
83. Noll, *America's God*, 307.
84. Nathan O. Hatch, *The Democratization of American Christianity* (New Haven: Yale University Press, 1989), 5.
85. Noll, *America's God*, 281, 296, 308.
86. Charles G. Finney, *Sermons on Important Subjects*, 3rd ed. (New York: John S. Taylor, 1836), 22, 24, 27, 29.
87. Although some scholars do not consider him a revivalist, Dwight had a great influence on Lyman Beecher and the Second Great Awakening. For information on Eli Todd, see W. H. Rockwell, "Biographical Sketch of the Late Eli Todd, M.D.," *U.S. Medical and Surgical Journal* 14 (1836): 173–74.
88. *The Diaries of Julia Cowles: A Connecticut Record, 1797–1803*, ed. Laura Hadley Moseley (New Haven: Yale University Press, 1931), 71. For an eighteenth-century example, see Thomas Kidd, "The Healing of Mercy Wheeler: Illness and Miracles among Early American Evangelicals," *William and Mary Quarterly* 63 (January 2006): 149–70.
89. Boyd Hilton analyzes the social and economic influences in nineteenth-century Britain among the elite of the Anglican Church of England and the Presbyterian Kirk of Scotland. Similarly to American evangelicalism, he found that that they oscillated between "optimism and pessimism, uncertain whether happiness or misery best testified to God's efficient governance." Moderate British evangelicals regarded pain as an essential part of the journey from sin to grace and as promoting discipline, while extreme evangelicals saw pain as a disturbance of God's order and tended toward resignation. Boyd Hilton, *Age of Atonement: The Influence of Evangelicalism on Social and Economic Thought, 1795–1865* (Oxford: Clarendon Press, 1988), 822, 11.
90. Nancy F. Cott, "Young Women in the Second Great Awakening in New England," *Feminist Studies* 3 (Autumn 1975): 16–18. Harrison Parker, *Hawley, Massachusetts: The First Fifty Years, 1770–1820* (Amherst, MA: Sara Publishing, 1992), 280–81.
91. Sophronia Grout, diary 1816–37 (hereafter S. Grout diary), microfilm, July 14, 1816, Pocumtuck Memorial Valley Association, Deerfield, MA (PVMA).
92. S. Grout diary, September 1816 and March 2, 1825.
93. Jonathan Grout, *The Substance of a Discourse Delivered at Conway, July 14, 1817, on the Occasion of the Interment of the Remains of Consider Wilder and Increase Biggs, Two Young Men Who Were Drowned in the Deerfield River on the 12th of the Same Month* (Northampton, MA: Thomas W. Shepard & Co.: 1817), 19–20.
94. S. Grout diary, June (year unknown).
95. Esther did not go to Saratoga Springs to find a cure but to seek relief. The first

advocates for hydropathy or water cure in the United States were Joel Shew and Russell Trall in the 1840s; Fuller, *Alternative Medicine*, 26. Esther Grout, diary, 1830–35 (hereafter E. Grout diary) microfilm, May 30, 1830 and June 12, 1830, PVMA.
96. E. Grout diary, February 16, 1834.
97. A Dr. Charles Knowlton practiced medicine in Hawley from 1824 to approximately 1830. However, he left town after sparking a theological split among the townspeople due to his advocacy of materialism and his wish to publish a book on his philosophy. The Reverend Grout attempted to dissuade Knowlton from publishing the controversial text if for no other reason than it was against the law. When Knowlton replied that he didn't care about any law, Grout retorted that laws were made for people who didn't care about them. Since Grout and his assistant pastor were in opposition to Knowlton's ideas, even going so far as enjoining their followers not to consult him for medical treatment, it seems unlikely that either daughter would have been under Knowlton's care. See *History of the Town of Ashfield, Franklin County, Massachusetts: From Its Settlement in 1742 until 1910* (Ashfield, MA: by town, 1910), 365, 368; and William Giles Atkins, *History of the Town of Hawley, Massachusetts, Franklin County, Massachusetts: From Its Settlement in 1771 until 1887; With Family Records and Biographical Sketches* (West Cummington, MA: By author, 1887), 91–92.
98. Atkins, *History of the Town of Hawley*, 92. That Moses Smith practiced allopathic medicine can be shown by the announcement that he had become a fellow of the Massachusetts Medical Society in 1833. "Other 6: No Title," *Massachusetts Medical Society, Medical Communications (1790–1913)*, vol. 5 (Boston: American Periodicals Series II, 1836), a90.
99. E. Grout diary, February 16, 1834.
100. Fuller, *Alternative Medicine*, 20–21. Also see Joseph F. Kett, *The Formation of the American Medical Profession: The Role of Institutions, 1780–1860* (New Haven: Yale University Press, 1968), 129. Fuller and Kett depend on information from Whitney Cross, *The Burned-Over District: The Social and Intellectual History of Enthusiastic Religion in Western New York, 1800–1850* (Ithaca, NY: Cornell University Press, 1950), 287, as well as comments from Samuel Thomson. Thomson abandoned farming and began an itinerant medical practice in New Hampshire, Maine, and Massachusetts in 1805. Cowles diary dates 1797–1803. John S. Haller, *The People's Doctor: Samuel Thomson and the American Botanical Movement, 1790–1860* (Carbondale: Southern Illinois University Press, 2000), 15.
101. As quoted in Ronald J. Zboray and Mary Saracino Zboray, *Everyday Ideas: Socioliterary Experience among Antebellum New Englanders* (Knoxville: University of Tennessee Press, 2006), 211.
102. Robert A. Gross provided a helpful framework for this discussion.
103. Fuller, *Alternative Medicine*, 18.
104. Robert Ferguson writes that reason, providence, and nature could be simultaneously central to the belief systems in men such as Thomas Jefferson, the emblem of

enlightened reason. "Jefferson can be a sincere Christian in a letter of 1803 to Benjamin Rush and then can dismiss the virgin birth, the divinity of Christ . . . when writing to William Short in 1819." Robert Ferguson, *The American Enlightenment, 1750–1820* (Cambridge: Harvard University Press, 1997), 77.

105. Catherine Albanese, *Nature Religion in America: From the Algonkin Indians to New Age* (Chicago: University of Chicago Press, 1990), 123–26.

5. MEDICINE AND MALPRACTICE

1. "Prosecution for Malpractice," *Boston Medical and Surgical Journal* (hereafter *BMSJ*) 30, no. 17 (May 29, 1844): 344.
2. DeVille used published reports of cases decided in appellate courts of various states, which do not constitute a complete record or predict the number of malpractice cases at the trial-court level. As DeVille stated, "ultimately, smaller scale studies of individual states may be warranted," but a systematic investigation of surviving trial records would require a search of hundreds of local courts. Kenneth DeVille, *Medical Malpractice in Nineteenth-Century America: Origins and Legacy* (New York: New York University Press, 1990), xii.
3. He compared increases in malpractice suits with increases in population. Between 1840 and 1880 the population increased 194 percent, while appellate malpractice decisions increased 1,228 percent, thus revealing that the increase in appellate decisions was not simply a function of population growth. DeVille, *Medical Malpractice*, 3, 26.
4. I identified cases through newspaper, LexisNexis Academic, and the *BSMJ* databases. See appendix C for a list of cases. The Court of Common Pleas dockets for the nineteenth century do not list physician or doctor in the names, so a researcher would need to know the names of doctors in order to limit the search. A systematic county-by-county search is possible but time-consuming, as a researcher would have to travel to each county seat. Some county records are on microfilm and others are not. This would be a fruitful exercise for a book on the topic.
5. Moses Mosman, account book, 1763–1820, vol. 1, June 8, 1771, and vol. 3, April 30, 1805, American Antiquarian Society, Worcester, MA.
6. It should be noted that American editions of early-nineteenth-century legal handbooks such as Joseph Chitty's *Practical Treatise on Pleading* (1812) suggested that lawyers could use either a writ of assumpsit (simple contract) or a writ of trespass on the case for malpractice suits. William Blackstone, Esq., *Commentaries on the Laws of England*, vol. 3 (Oxford: Clarendon Press, 1765), 122. DeVille, *Medical Malpractice*, 157–59, 165.
7. Morton Horwitz, *The Transformation of American Law, 1780–1860* (New York: Oxford University Press, 1992), 85.
8. Caution must be exercised when applying these characterizations of churches and their functions in conflict resolution to other regions of the country; Nelson found his evidence in Massachusetts. Nelson, *Dispute and Conflict Resolution*, 4, 23, 26, 36.

9. The expansion of commerce and the spread of religious dissent were not the only impetuses for change; Nelson cites the institutionalization of partisan politics as a possible explanation as well, although he qualifies such a connection: "it is impossible to analyze the relationship between political conflict and the rate of litigation with the same precision with which the litigation rate could be related to commercial growth or even to the spread of religious dissent." William E. Nelson, *Americanization of the Common Law: The Impact of Legal Change on Massachusetts Society, 1760–1830* (Cambridge: Harvard University Press, 1975), 122, 127, 132.
10. Poisoning, intentional and accidental, became a central topic of interest, specifically in cases involving druggists and apothecaries selling impure or dangerous substances. James C. Mohr, *Doctors and the Law: Medical Jurisprudence in Nineteenth-Century America* (Baltimore: Johns Hopkins University Press, 1993), 20–24, 44.
11. Ibid., 52, 69.
12. John J. Elwell, *A Medico-Legal Treatise, Medical Evidence, and Insanity, Compromising Elements of Medical Jurisprudence* (New York: J. S. Voorhies, 1860), 22.
13. Horwitz argues that in general (not just in respect to medical malpractice) "a gradual shift in emphasis from an older conception of failure to perform a duty to a distinctly modern emphasis on careless performance" occurred over the course of the nineteenth century. He locates a dominant emphasis on careless performance after the Civil War. Horwitz, *Transformation of American Law*, 88.
14. *McCandless v. McWha* 22 Penn. 261 (1853) as quoted in Elwell, *Medico-Legal Treatise*, 118, 128.
15. Alexander Young, "The Law of Malpractice," *BMSJ* 82, no. 23 (June 9, 1870): 435; Elwell, *Medico-Legal Treatise*, 125.
16. Elwell, *Medico-Legal Treatise*, 125–26.
17. *Brown v. Kendall*, 60 Mass. 292 LEXIS 150 (1850).
18. Elwell, *Medico-Legal Treatise*, 38–44.
19. Young, "The Law of Malpractice," 439–40.
20. DeVille, *Medical Malpractice*, 33.
21. Walter K. Manning, "Prosecution for Mal-practice," *BMSJ* 40, no. 16 (May 23, 1849): 318; Walter K. Manning, "Trial for Malpractice," *BMSJ* 42, no. 5 (February 27, 1850): 79; and "Case of Mal-practice," *BMSJ* 54, no. 6 (March 13, 1856): 111.
22. "News and Misc Items," *Boston Evening Transcript*, November 9, 1854, 1.
23. *Ashworth v. Kittridge* [no number in original], 66 Mass. 193 LEXIS 211 (October 1853) serves as one example of *BMSJ* articles being used by multiple newspapers. See "List of Massachusetts Cases Identified" in appendix C; DeVille, *Medical Malpractice*, 59.
24. "Another Suit of Mal-Practice," *BMSJ* 51, no. 25 (January 17, 1855): 504.
25. Mohr, *Doctors and the Law*, 114. "A deep pocket theory already existed," stated Allen D. Spiegel and Florence Kavaler in "America's First Medical Malpractice Crisis, 1835–1865," *Journal of Community Health* 22 (August 4, 1997): 301.
26. DeVille, *Medical Malpractice*, 43.
27. Horwitz, *Transformation of American Law*, 208, 28. Massachusetts under the legal

guidance of Chief Justice Shaw especially saw "corporate industrial interests" prevail "over lesser, private ones," according to Leonard W. Levy. Leonard W. Levy, *The Law of the Commonwealth and Chief Justice Shaw* (Cambridge: Harvard University Press, 1957), 332.
28. DeVille, *Medical Malpractice*, 7.
29. William Andrus Alcott, *The House I Live In; Or the Human Body* (Boston: Light & Stearns, 1837), as quoted in Michael Sappol, *A Traffic of Dead Bodies: Anatomy and Embodied Social Identity in Nineteenth-Century America* (Princeton: Princeton University Press, 2002), 178, 181.
30. DeVille, *Medical Malpractice*, 86; Hyman Kuritz, "The Popularization of Science in Nineteenth-Century America," *History of Education Quarterly* 21 (Autumn 1981): 262.
31. Sappol, *Traffic of Dead Bodies*, 192.
32. Calvin Cutter, *First Book on Anatomy, Physiology, and Hygiene: for Grammar Schools and Families: with Eighty-eight Engravings* (New York: Clark, Austin & Smith, 1861 ca. 1852), 21, 29, 30.
33. Lamar Riley Murphy, *Enter the Physician: The Transformation of Domestic Medicine, 1760–1860* (Tuscaloosa: University of Alabama Press, 1991), 167.
34. J. D. Mansfield, "Dr. Lambert's Popular Anatomy and Physiology—Quackery, &c.," *BMSJ* 42, no. 12 (April 24, 1850): 249.
35. "Practical Schools of Anatomy," *BMSJ* 39, no. 9 (September 27, 1848): 187.
36. DeVille, *Medical Malpractice*, 157.
37. "Prosecution of Mal-Practice," *BMSJ* 48, no. 14 (May 4, 1853): 281–83, and "Cases of Mal-Practice Tried in the Supreme Court at Cambridge," *BMSJ* 54, no. 6 (March 13, 1856): 109. The case eventually went before the Massachusetts Supreme Court in October 1853. The defendant filed for exceptions and challenged the verdict based on improper testimony. The plaintiff's attorney had read medical texts into testimony over objections by the defendant's counsel, and the Supreme Court ruled that, because a medical text could not be cross-examined, it was improper. The Supreme Court sustained the exceptions and a new trial was ordered. *Ashworth v. Kittridge*, 66 Mass. 193 LEXIS 211 (October, 1853).
38. The phrase "enough to puzzle a Philadelphia lawyer" was a common expression in the Early Republic, used in speaking of a difficult point. Bartlett J. Whiting, *Early American Proverbs and Proverbial Sayings* (Cambridge: Harvard University Press, 1978), 334. "Prosecutions for Mal-practice," *BMSJ* 51, no. 15 (November 8, 1854): 305.
39. DeVille, *Medical Malpractice*, 61.
40. "Medical Paragraphs," *Boston Post*, August 4, 1856, 2.
41. Horwitz, *Transformation of American Law*, xv, 5, 30, 21.
42. Levy, *Law of Commonwealth*, 166, 168.
43. Horwitz, *Transformation of American Law*, 209–10. Another landmark case showing the belief that verdicts should protect societal interests rather than those of individuals can be seen in *Charles River Bridge v. Warren Bridge*, 36 U.S. 420 (1837), in which the "Charles River Bridge case offered a convenient opportunity

to create a legal covering for public policy choices favoring technological innovation and economic change." Stanley I. Kutler, *Privilege and Creative Destruction: The Charles River Bridge Case* (Baltimore: Johns Hopkins University Press, 1971), 161.

44. Some debate exists over the relationship between extralegal forces in society and the development of legal doctrine. Traditional legal historians view legal doctrine as developing autonomously from outside social influences. Legal historians such as Lawrence Friedman depict legal doctrine as a function wholly dependent on social factors such as economic interests and politics. Horwitz articulates what historian Jefferson White calls a "filter assumption," in which legal doctrine is seen as a product of economic and political ideas filtered through legal ideas and theories. White does not disagree with Horwitz's "filter assumption" but argues that changes in legal doctrine seldom happen in the systematic way that Horwitz describes. Instead, legal change usually occurs as a salient change; it continues to operate from an earlier period, but salience varies depending on the area of law. I rely on Horwitz's work because I agree with his holistic approach, in which interconnections between social, economic, political, and legal institutions exist. Jefferson White, "Representing Change in Early American Law: An Alternative to Horwitz's Approach," in *The Law in America, 1607–1861,* ed. William Pencak and Wythe W. Holt, Jr. (New York: The New-York Historical Society, 1989), 240–41, 250–51.

45. Horwitz, *Transformation of American Law,* 30, 23.
46. "Surgeon Protected by Contract," *BMSJ* 48, no. 23 (July 6, 1853): 465.
47. Nelson, *Americanization of the Common Law,* 21, 150. Horwitz, *Transformation of American Law,* 28.
48. *Commonwealth v. Thompson* [sic] 6 Mass. 134 (1809), as quoted in Alexander Young, "The Law of Malpractice—Part II," *BMSJ* 84, no. 1 (January 5, 1871): 5–6.
49. *Rex v. Spiller;* 1 Lewin 181; *Rex v. Webb,* 1 Moody & Robinson, 405, as cited by Young, "The Law of Malpractice, Part II," 8.
50. Young, "The Law of Malpractice, Part II," 1, 7, 12.
51. "No Headline," *Springfield Republican,* April 21, 1866, 1; and "Items," *Boston Daily Journal,* April 21, 1866, 2.
52. See a sample of "Criminal Cases in Massachusetts" (appendix D). This is by no means an exhaustive list of announcements in Massachusetts newspapers; that would require a more systematic review.
53. Young, "The Law of Malpractice, Part II," 7. DeVille, *Medical Malpractice,* 165–66.
54. Horwitz, *Transformation of American Law,* 87.
55. Mohr, *Doctors and the Law,* 112, and chapter 3 of this book.

CONCLUSION

1. Paul Starr, *The Social Transformation of American Medicine* (New York: Basic Books,

1982); Charles H. Rosenberg, *The Care of Strangers: The Rise of America's Hospital System* (New York: Basic Books, 1987); and Samuel Haber, *The Quest for Authority and Honor in American Professions, 1750–1900* (Chicago: Chicago University Press, 1991) are some famous examples.
2. Starr, *Social Transformation*, 81, 102, 110, 120–22, 129.
3. Starr further distinguishes his study by differentiating between social and cultural authority. Social authority involves the control of actions through commands, whereas cultural authority "entails the construction of reality through definitions of fact and value." Starr focuses on cultural authority. Starr, *Social Transformation*, 13, 17, 129.
4. Ibid., 135–36.
5. Nancy Tomes, *The Gospel of Germs: Men, Women, and the Microbe in American Life* (Cambridge: Harvard University Press, 1998), 13.
6. Ibid., 6.

INDEX

account books: farming, 50–51; medical, 3–4, 10–13, 26, 44, 51
advertisements, for drugs, 5, 25, 33, 35–39, 111, 165n23
Alcott, A. Bronson, 83–85
Alcott, Louisa May, 84–85
Alcott, William A., 102–3
American Medical Association, 3, 115
Ashburnham, Massachusetts, 12, 14

Beck, Theodric R., 95
Beecher, Lyman, 85–86
Bigelow, Henry J., 46
Bigelow, Jacob, 26–27
Blackstone, Sir William, 94
bleeding, 1–2, 4, 10–17, 20, 117–23, 125, 137–38; forms of, 14,-15, 158n22. *See also* leeches
Boerhaave, Herman, 2, 155n3
Boston, Massachusetts, 3–4, 13, 28, 34, 41, 43, 46, 50, 52, 56, 59, 61, 65, 83; churches of, 75–79; medical practice in, 11–13, 22, 26–28; newspapers of, 35; physicians in, 10–11, 14, 19, 26, 52–53, 55, 72, 100, 105, 109
Boston Dispensary, 27, 62–63, 65–66
Boston Medical and Surgical Journal, 28, 57–58, 61, 92, 95, 97, 104, 107, 135, 149–50
Brigham, Anna Sophia, 69

Brigham, Joseph, 51–52
Brown, John, 2, 25, 155n3
Buchan, William, 22, 34, 161n55
Buckminster, Joseph, 77

calomel, 2, 5, 10–13, 17–18, 20, 26, 29–31, 42, 44, 73, 119–26, 138, 157n8, 166n40
Calvinism, 70, 76, 81, 85
cathartics, 5, 12–13, 16–23, 26, 29–31, 35, 42, 45, 47–48, 70, 108, 117–26, 137–38, 160n36, 161n54
Chandler, George, 19, 22–23, 31
Chandler, J. L., 61
Channing, William Ellery, 77, 80, 174n47
Chase, Lucy, 79, 81, 90
Chauncy, Charles, 76–77
Child, Daniel, 29, 44, 78–79, 81, 90–91
Child, Lydia Maria, 43
common law, English, 94, 108
Congregationalism, 6, 68, 74–75, 81, 85–86, 90, 114
Cowles, Julia, 86, 89
Cullen, William, 2, 155n3
cure, 2, 6, 15, 24, 26, 34–35, 37–39, 42, 47, 66–67, 75, 78–89, 91–92, 97, 100, 108, 111, 114; language of, 7–8, 68–72
Cutter, Calvin, 103–4
Dall, Caroline, 82–83
Deerfield, Massachusetts, 3–4, 12–13;

Deerfield, Massachusetts, (*continued*)
  medical practice in, 11, 14, 26–27; physicians in, 13, 56
Dickenson, Rebecca, 69–70
diet, 2, 6, 12, 20, 42, 44, 157n8; vegetarian, 19
diseases. *See* illnesses
domestic remedies. *See* home remedies
Dorsey, John Syng, 69
Dwight, Timothy, 85–86, 177n87

economic exchange systems: local exchange, 50–52, 54–58, 60, 114; long-distance trade, 50–52, 56–57, 60, 63, 114
Elwell, John J., 96–98, 110
Emerson, Ralph Waldo, 81–82
emetics, 5, 13, 20–21, 23, 26, 37, 44, 73, 75, 108, 117–22, 124–25, 127–29, 137–38, 161n48, 161n62
empiricism, 2, 10, 36, 59, 156n4, 167n50

Finney, Charles, 85–86
First Great Awakening, 76
Fiske, Deborah, 15, 21, 75–76, 86, 91
Flint, Edward, 52–54, 60, 131
Forward, Justus, 68–69, 171n6
Fuller, Margaret, 82

galvanism, 78–79
Gay, Ebenezer, 76–77
Geist, Christian F., 83, 176n77
Grout, Esther, 88–90, 178n95
Grout, Jonathan, 87, 178n97
Grout, Sophronia, 87–90

Hartshorn, John, 19, 30
Harvard University, 75, 77; divinity school, 81; medical school, 3, 22, 27
health journals, popular, 6, 16, 19–20, 103, 111; *The American Frugal Housewife*, 43; *Domestic Duties*, 63; *Domestic Medicine*, 22; *Hall's Journal of Health*, 20; *Ladies' Home Magazine*, 20; *Medical Admonitions*, 15; *The Physiological Family Physician*, 103; *Popular Anatomy and Physiology*, 104; *Primary Physiology for Schools*, 103; *The Treasure of Health*, 34

Heath, Mary, 80–81
Heaton, Hannah, 70
heroic depletive therapy, 1–3, 5, 9–12, 14, 16, 18, 20, 26, 31–32, 48, 70, 90, 115, 125, 157n8, 159n25
Heywood, Benjamin F., 55
Hodge, Hugh Lenox, 45, 69
homeopathy. *See under* medical practice, alternative
home remedies, 33–36. *See also* self-medication
Hooker, Worthington, 28–30, 36, 46, 113

illnesses: chronic diarrhea, 6, 37, 42, 48; constipation, 5, 18–20, 30–32, 34, 42, 47, 64, 116; consumption (tuberculosis), 45, 75, 116; dysentery, 6, 41–42; dyspepsia, 6, 37, 41–42, 44; epidemics, 4, 6; gastrointestinal, 4, 18–20, 42; general fevers, 4, 14–16, 19, 40–42, 48, 73, 95, 98; gout, 25; inflammation, 14–16, 31, 42, 48, 64, 109–10; respiratory, 21, 40; rheumatism, 4, 25, 34, 45, 47, 64, 98; scarlet fever, 46, 83; typhoid, 6, 116; typhus, 6, 11, 41; wounds, 4, 42–43, 105; yellow fever, 1, 31. *See also appendix B*
industrialization: accidents of, 92, 107, 115; age of, 8, 43, 65, 114; tort cases during, 102, 106; workers of, 101, 111

Jackson, James, Sr., 11, 27, 43, 46, 65, 72, 76
Jarvis, Edward, 103–4

Lambert, Thomas, 103–4
lawsuits, medical. *See* malpractice
lawsuits, non-medical: doctrine of "assumption of risk," 107; *Farwell v. Boston and Worcester R.R.*, 106–7; fellow-servant rule, 106; industrial torts, 102; public policy of, 8, 107, 181n43; role of judges in, 106; "trespass, upon the case," 94; writ of trespass, 94
leeches, 14–16, 31, 83, 138
Lowe, Abraham, 12–15, 18, 20, 25–26, 31, 119, 125–26
Lowell, Mary Gardiner, 11, 34, 47

· Index · 187

malpractice, 7–8, 92–98, 114–15; appellate cases of, 7, 93, 100–101, 106, 179n2; criminal cases of, 108–10; definition of, 93; in Massachusetts, 93, 99, 101, 105; negligence in, 7–8, 23, 92, 94, 96–98, 101, 106, 109–12; nonsurgical cases of, 97; nuisance in, 7, 92, 94, 115; as public policy, 8, 107, 181n43

Massachusetts General Hospital, 4, 6, 11, 13, 27, 29, 40, 62–63, 65, 99, 101; admission process of, 62; hospital records of, 5–6, 33, 39, 48; occupation classification of patients in, 134; patients of, 21, 34–35, 41, 47, 50; physicians of, 11, 43–46, 100; treatments of, 10, 14–15, 17, 20, 22, 42–43, 47. *See also appendixes A and B*

Massachusetts Medical Society, 13, 27–28

Mayhew, Jonathan, 76–77

medical practice, alternative: botanic, 61, 84, 108, 156n9; homeopathy, 10, 16, 46, 79, 83–84, 176n74; mesmerism, 61; Thomsonian, 10, 46, 89, 167n49, 170n37; water cure, 83–84, 114, 167n49

medical practice, regular: expectant, 2, 10–12, 14, 17–18, 24, 26–29, 156n8; heroic depletive (*see* heroic depletive therapy); rural, 4, 11, 14, 28–29, 50–52, 54–58, 61, 66, 89; urban, 4, 8, 11, 26–29, 49–52, 54–55, 59, 65–66

medical procedures: blister, 17, 31, 69, 73, 83, 119, 120, 122; delivery of baby, 117–18, 122, 149, 152; purges, 4, 31; pukes, 4, 20, 31. *See also* bleeding

Merlin, Lewis, 34, 43, 163n2

Metcalf, John G., 58–60, 133

Mosman, Moses, 4, 12, 14, 18, 20, 22, 25–26, 31, 52–53, 55, 60, 93, 117–18, 125–26, 130

opiates, 13, 21–23, 31, 79, 121–25, 128, 161n55; camphor, 22, 117–19, 122, 124; laudanum, 23–25, 161n60; narcotics, 12, 22–23, 30–31, 47–48, 137–38, 161n54; paregoric elixir, 22, 118–19, 122–23

Paige, A., 78–70, 175n53

pain management, 5, 14, 21–24, 30–34, 38, 75, 84; palliative, 3, 24; perception of, 68–71, 74, 78, 90; and sedatives, 23–24. *See also* opiates

Park, Louisa, 72–73, 90

Park, John, 72, 90

Parker, Theodore, 82, 176n68

Parkinson, James, 15, 41

patent medicines, 33, 37, 57, 115; Anderson's Scots Pills, 35; Bateman's Pectoral Drops, 35; British Oil, 35; Daffy's Elixir Salutis, 35; Dalby's Carminative, 35; Dover's Powder, 57; Dr. Glauber's Salts, 45; Dr. Gordak's Jelly of Pomegranate and Peruvian Pills, 37–38; Godfrey's Cordial, 35; Dr. Hill's Pills, 45; Dr. Jackson's Pile Embrocation, 36; Dr. James's Powder, 45, 57; Dr. Jones' Pill, 45; Dr. Relfe's Botanical Drops, 35; Herrick's Kid Strengthening Plasters, 38–39; Hopper's Female Pills, 35, 57; Johnson's Pill, 57; Steer's Opodeldoc, 35, 45; Turlington's Balsam of Life, 35

patients: age of, 6, 22, 40, 65; class of, 6, 20, 35, 40, 44, 61–62, 73, 79; gender of, 6, 64–65, 97; historical study of, 3–4; marital status of, 6, 60, 64, 87, 134; nationality of, 6; occupation of, 66–67, 134; poverty of, 58–59. *See also* self-medication

payment methods: banknotes, 57; barter, 6, 49, 51, 63–64; cash, 5–6, 8, 49–63, 65–66, 110, 114, 130–32, 153; credit, 6, 50, 53, 55–56, 58, 60, 62, 66, 114, 153; promissory notes, 8, 49–53, 55–56, 58–60, 62, 66, 93, 114, 130–32; social credit, 6, 49–50, 63–66, 114

Peabody, Elizabeth, 46, 82

Pierce, John, 80–81

Philadelphia, 2, 10, 25, 41, 43, 69, 95, 105, 157n8

physicians, orthodox, 2–5, 13–17, 20, 32–33, 45, 61, 68, 76, 79, 81, 89, 100, 103; definition of, 156n9

physicians, unorthodox, 4–5, 33, 45–46, 89, 90; definition of, 156n9

Porter, Jacob, 17, 21, 23, 30–31, 36, 44, 71–72

providence: general, 74; miracles, 74; special, 6, 68, 74, 78, 81, 86, 90

quackery: advertisements of, 36; attitudes toward, 45–46, 79; definition of, 166n47; practitioners of, 45, 61, 84; remedies of, 39, 44–45, 57

religious beliefs. *See* Calvinism; Congregationalism; Revivalism; Transcendentalism; Unitarianism
Revivalism, 7, 68, 85–90
Richardson, Experience, 70
Rush, Benjamin, 1–2, 9–10, 14, 17, 25, 31–32, 155n3, 160n30, 163n99

Saltonstall, Nathaniel, 53
Sargent, Joseph, 11, 15–16, 19, 23, 30–31, 45
Seaton, Ambrose, 22, 37
Second Great Awakening, 85
self-medication, 5–6, 33, 39–40, 42, 44, 47, 137
Shaw, Chief Justice Lemuel, 107, 181n27
Snow, Caleb, 13–14, 18, 20, 26–28, 31, 55, 58, 60, 124, 126, 159n25
social reform, 85, 87; antislavery, 86, 174n47, 176n68; health, 86, 91; hygiene, 102–4; temperance, 20, 86

Sprague, John, 52
Sudbury, Massachusetts, 12, 14, 52, 70, 93
Swain, William, 38

Taylor, Amos, 56
Thomson, Samuel, 108–9, 156n4, 178n100
Thomsonism. *See under* medical practice, alternative
Transcendentalism, 7, 68, 81–85, 90–91

Unitarianism, 7, 68, 76–81, 85, 90, 114; on abolition, 174n47

Ware, John, 22
Wessellhoeft, William, 79
White, Caroline Barrett, 23–24
Williams, Stephen West, 13–16, 18–22, 26–29, 31, 55, 57, 123, 125–26, 160n36, 162n84
Williams, William Stoddard, 4, 13–15, 18, 20, 22, 26, 31, 56, 57, 120–27, 132, 159n25
Woodworth, Francis C., 9
Worcester, Massachusetts, 3–4, 54, 67, 79; medical practice in, 11–12, 55; physicians in, 11–12, 52–53, 55, 58